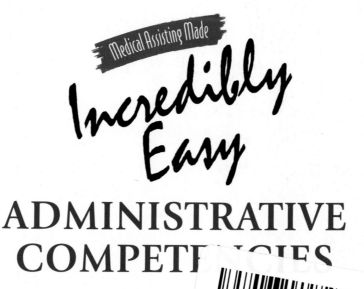

Medical Assisting Made

Incredibly Easy

ADMINISTRATIVE
COMPETENCIES

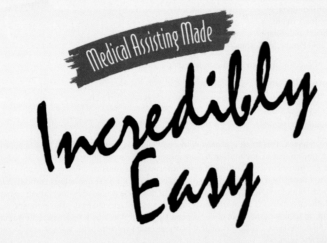

Medical Assisting Made

Incredibly Easy

ADMINISTRATIVE COMPETENCIES

Geri Kale-Smith, MS, CMA

Medical Office Administration Programs

William Rainey Harper College

Palatine, Illinois

Wolters Kluwer | Lippincott Williams & Wilkins
Health

Philadelphia • Baltimore • New York • London
Buenos Aires • Hong Kong • Sydney • Tokyo

Executive Editor: John Goucher
Senior Managing Editor: Rebecca Kerins
Marketing Manager: Hilary Henderson
Production Editor: Eve Malakoff-Klein
Illustrator: Bot Roda
Designer: Joan Wendt
Compositor: Circle Graphics, Inc.
Printer: R.R. Donnelley & Sons—Crawfordsville

9 8 7 6 5 4 3 2 1

Library of Congress Cataloging-in-Publication Data

Kale-Smith, Geri.
  Administrative competencies / Geri Kale-Smith.
    p. ; cm. — (Medical assisting made incredibly easy)
  Includes index.
  ISBN-13: 978-0-7817-7810-7
  ISBN-10: 0-7817-7810-7
  1. Medical assistants. 2. Medical offices. I. Title. II. Series.
  [DNLM: 1. Practice Management, Medical. 2. Allied Health Personnel. 3. Medical Sec-
retaries. W 80 K14a 2008]
  R728.8.K35 2008
  610.73'7069—dc22

                              2007001966

DISCLAIMER

Care has been taken to confirm the accuracy of the information present and to describe generally accepted practices. However, the authors, editors, and publisher are not responsible for
errors or omissions or for any consequences from application of the information in this book
and make no warranty, expressed or implied, with respect to the currency, completeness, or accuracy of the contents of the publication. Application of this information in a particular situation
remains the professional responsibility of the practitioner; the clinical treatments described and
recommended may not be considered absolute and universal recommendations.

The authors, editors, and publisher have exerted every effort to ensure that drug selection
and dosage set forth in this text are in accordance with the current recommendations and
practice at the time of publication. However, in view of ongoing research, changes in government regulations, and the constant flow of information relating to drug therapy and drug reactions, the reader is urged to check the package insert for each drug for any change in
indications and dosage and for added warnings and precautions. This is particularly important when the recommended agent is a new or infrequently employed drug.

Some drugs and medical devices presented in this publication have Food and Drug Administration (FDA) clearance for limited use in restricted research settings. It is the responsibility
of the health care provider to ascertain the FDA status of each drug or device planned for use
in their clinical practice.

To purchase additional copies of this book, call our customer service department at **(800) 638-
3030** or fax orders to **(301) 223-2320**. International customers should call **(301) 223-2300**.

Visit Lippincott Williams & Wilkins on the Internet: http://www.lww.com. Lippincott Williams
& Wilkins customer service representatives are available from 8:30 am to 6:00 p.m., EST.

PREFACE

Medical Assisting Made Incredibly Easy is an exciting new series designed to make learning enjoyable for medical assisting students. Each book in the series uses a light-hearted, humorous approach to presenting information. Maria, a Certified Medical Assistant, guides students through the books, offering helpful tips and insights along the way.

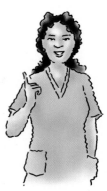

Medical Assisting Made Incredibly Easy takes a practical approach, providing students with the critical information that they need to know, including complete coverage of the core skills they must master in their studies. The series covers all competencies based on the standards and guidelines established for medical assisting by the Commission on Accreditation of Allied Health Educational Programs (CAAHEP) and the Accrediting Bureau of Health Education Schools (ABHES).

ABOUT THIS BOOK

Medical Assisting Made Incredibly Easy: Administrative Competencies provides instruction in CAAHEP's administrative and general competencies, as well as ABHES's competencies related to administrative duties, professionalism, communication, legal concepts, office management, instruction, and financial management. These are among the skills that students must master to pass the test required to become either a Certified Medical Assistant or a Registered Medical Assistant.

HOW THIS BOOK IS ORGANIZED

Medical Assisting Made Incredibly Easy: Administrative Competencies is designed to be enjoyable to read, as well as highly informative. The book is divided into two parts:

- Part One, which includes chapters 1 to 3, covers general skills, such as communication, law and ethics, and operational functions.
- Part Two, which includes chapters 4 to 8, covers administrative skills, such as managing appointments, documentation, and medical coding.

SPECIAL FEATURES

Each chapter in this book includes special features designed to guide students in their study. These elements will help students to identify the most important information in the chapter and to understand all of it.

- **Chapter Checklist** *Chapter Checklist* includes a list of skills and other important information that students will gain after reading the material.

- **Closer Look** *Closer Look* explores chapter information in more detail in a list or summary form.

- **Running Smoothly** *Running Smoothly* features situations that medical assistants may encounter in a medical office and shows how students can apply what they have learned to those situations.

- **Ask the Professional** *Ask the Professional* offers expert advice on how to handle difficult situations that medical assistants may face in the workplace.

- **Secrets for Success** *Secrets for Success* provides tips for studying, for remembering important material, and for success in a career as a medical assistant.

- **Legal Brief** *Legal Brief* provides important legal and ethical information, including how the Health Insurance Portability and Accountability Act (HIPAA) impacts medical assisting.

- **Word to the Wise** *Word to the Wise* covers terminology that students might find challenging, providing a definition and pronunciation for each term.

- **Hands On** *Hands On* contains procedures for important skills and tasks.

- **Chapter Highlights** *Chapter Highlights* summarizes a chapter's key content.

In addition to the above features, this book also includes bolded key terms throughout each chapter and a Glossary in the back of the book, as well as many other boxed features and tables.

ADDITIONAL RESOURCES

In addition to the text, the following resources are available for students and instructors:

- *Study Guide for Medical Assisting Made Incredibly Easy: Administrative Competencies* includes learning activities and exercises, quizzes, puzzles, certification review questions, and competency evaluation forms so students can practice their skills and measure their success.

- An **Online Course** provides interactive exercises and review opportunities that support the text and classroom experience.

- An **Instructor's Resource CD-ROM** with test generator, PowerPoint slides, image bank, answers to study guide questions, and customizable competency evaluation forms helps instructors optimize their teaching. The Instructor's Resource CD-ROM also includes information on where in the book and Study Guide each ABHES and CAAHEP competency is covered.

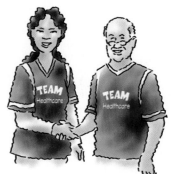

- A complete set of **Lesson Plans** is also available to instructors.

Medical Assisting Made Incredibly Easy: Administrative Competencies is designed to make the study of medical assisting fun and effective. The purpose of this book, and the entire *Medical Assisting Made Incredibly Easy* series, is student success!

USER'S GUIDE

Hello, my name is Maria. I'm a Certified Medical Assistant and educator, as well as your guide through this textbook. There are a number of features in this **Medical Assisting Made Incredibly Easy** text to help you learn everything you need to become a successful medical assistant. Read through this User's Guide to orient yourself to everything the text has to offer. Good luck in your medical assisting studies!

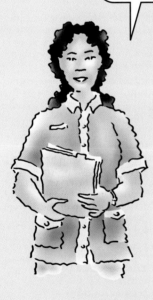

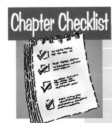

Chapter Checklist

- Describe the two main branches of the American legal system
- Identify the three parts of a contract
- Explain the difference between implied contracts and expressed contracts
- List the items that must appear in a contract termination letter
- Explain informed consent, who may sign a consent form, and under what conditions informed consent cannot be given
- Describe the importance of the medical record as a legal document
- Identify and respond to issues of confidentiality
- Demonstrate knowledge of federal and state health care legislation and regulations
- Summarize the reasons for lawsuits against medical professionals and identify three possible defenses
- Explain the ways in which medical law applies to the medical assistant
- Identify the main ethical principles and issues in health care
- Perform within legal and ethical boundaries

Chapter Checklists orient you to the material that's covered in the current chapter.

Closer Look — THE PATIENT APPOINTMENT BOOK

The reduced-size page at right shows patient appointments for one day in an office with three physicians.

- Notice that there is a column for each physician, plus a column for patients scheduled for blood tests in the lab.
- The matrix shows that Dr. Jones doesn't come in until 9:00 A.M. on Tuesdays. Dr. Stowe spends the morning seeing patients who are in the hospital. Dr. Jones goes to lunch at noon and the lab is closed for lunch between 1:00 P.M. and 2:00 P.M.

Closer Look boxes explore topics in more detail.

Running Smoothly — KEEPING RECORDS CURRENT

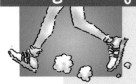

Running Smoothly boxes feature situations that you may encounter in a medical office and teach you to apply what you've learned to those situations.

How do you identify and remove the charts of inactive patients from the active records files?

The Hands On feature on page 186 tells you to put a year label on the folder when you create a chart for a new patient. Taking this step allows you to keep the active charts in the files separate from the inactive ones. Here's how.

- Each time an established patient visits the office, check the year label on his chart.
- If the year label is not for the current year, replace it with the current year's label.
- At the end of each year, go through the medical records and remove the charts of all patients whose year labels are older than the limit the office sets for active patients. For example, if the office requires that a patient must have been seen within the past year to remain active, you would remove all charts that don't have this year's label on them. Since you put new labels on the charts of ⌐⌐⌐ in during the year, none of their ⌐⌐⌐.

⌐⌐⌐-year time limit for active patients, ⌐⌐⌐ charts from the active files that ⌐⌐⌐ than five years old. Some offices ⌐⌐⌐ time limit. Always check your ⌐⌐⌐emoving any charts.

Ask the Professional — MANAGING APPOINTMENTS

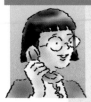

Q: *A patient called the office last week and asked for an appointment next Monday at 1:00 P.M. Another patient was already scheduled then for a complete physical examination. But the caller said he could only come at 1:00, so I gave him the appointment anyway. Now the physician has to work this patient in. How could I have handled this situation better?*

A: It's your job to control the appointment schedule. You should have politely but firmly explained that 1:00 was already taken. You could have offered the patient another time on Monday or a 1:00 appointment on another day of the week. You also could have offered to put him on the "move-up" list if there is a cancellation for the time he wants. Remember, YOU control the schedule. Don't ever let it control you!

Ask the Professional boxes offer expert advice on how to handle difficult situations that you may face in the workplace.

Secrets for Success 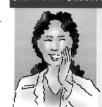 **CHART ORGANIZATION**

Here's a tip to help you recall the two main ways charts are organized.

- Remember that *P* stands for *problem*. In a POMR, records are organized around each medical *problem*.
- Remember that *S* stands for *source*. In an SOMR, records of the same type or *source*—such as x-ray results—are grouped together.

Secrets for Success boxes provide tips for studying, for remembering important material, and for success in your career as a medical assistant.

Legal Brief 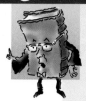 **QUALITY IMPROVEMENT AND HIPAA**

HIPAA was passed to:

- set standards for the security and privacy of patients' health information; these standards are covered in detail in other chapters of this book.
- set standards for submitting claims to patients' health insurers; you'll read about these standards in Chapter 8.

As with CLIA, medical offices need to have QI programs in place to make sure HIPAA standards are being met. For example, HIPAA requires that each medical office have a privacy officer. This person is responsible for seeing that patients' information is handled in the ways HIPAA requires.

Legal Briefs provide important legal and ethical information, including how the Health Insurance Portability and Accountability Act (HIPAA) affects your work in the medical office.

Word to the Wise 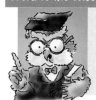 **res judicata** (rez YOO-dee-KAH-tuh)

Latin term that means "the thing has been decided"; this legal term means that once the lawsuit has been settled between the two parties, the losing party cannot sue the winner.

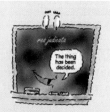

Word to the Wise boxes cover terminology that you might find challenging, providing a definition and pronunciation for each term.

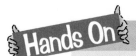 **USING THE ICD-9-CM**   7-1

Follow these steps to use the ICD-9-CM to code patient diagnoses.

1. Choose the main term in the diagnostic statement.
2. Locate the main term in the alphabetic index of Volume 2.
3. Refer to all notes and conventions under the main term.
4. Find the appropriate indented term under the main term.
5. Follow any indicated instructions, such as *see also*.
6. Confirm the code selected from the index by looking it up in Volume 1.
7. Add any fourth or fifth digits provided by Volume 1 as necessary.
8. Assign the code on the claim form.
9. Code the reason for the visit first. Then, code any other conditions that affect the patient's treatment for that visit.
   - Code a chronic condition as long as it applies to the patient's treatment.
   - Don't code a diagnosis that no longer applies.
10. Make sure an ICD-9 code is linked to each service or procedure provided to the patient.
    - For outpatient surgery, code the diagnosis that applies to the procedure.
    - If the postoperative diagnosis differs from the preoperative diagnosis, use the postoperative diagnosis.
11. Identify services for situations other than disease or injury, such as follow-up care, with the appropriate V-code.
    - List the V-code first, followed by the code for the condition.

Hands On boxes contain step-by-step, easy-to-follow procedures for important skills and tasks.

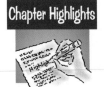 **Chapter Highlights**

- Patient charts are legal records that show the quality of patient care.
- Preparing and maintaining patient charts is an important responsibility.
- Understanding chart organization is important—in order to file items in charts properly and to write in charts correctly.
- All patients' contact with the office must be documented properly.
- Medical records files can be organized alphabetically or numerically.
- Charts are grouped into active, inactive, and closed categories.
- Computer technology is changing the way medical records are organized, maintained, and stored.

Chapter Highlights summarize a chapter's key content.

REVIEWERS

Julie Akason, BSN, MAEd
College of St. Catherine
St. Paul, Minnesota

Nina Beaman, MS, BA, AAS
Bryant and Stratton College
Richmond, Virginia

Michelle Buchman, RN, BSN, BC
St. John's Marian Center
Springfield, Missouri

Tracie Fuqua, BS
Wallace State Community College
Hanceville, Alabama

Robyn Gohsman, AAS
Medical Careers Institute
Newport News, Virginia

Christine Golden, MS, MT (ASCP)
Waukesha County Technical College
Pewaukee, Wisconsin

Rebecca Hickey, RN, RMC, AHI, CHI, BA
Butler Technology and Career Development Schools
Fairfield Township, Ohio

Joanna Holly, RN, BS, MS
Midstate College
Peoria, Illinois

Dorothy Kiel, BS
Rhodes State College
Lima, Ohio

Carol Lacy, RN, BSN, PHN
College of Marin
Novato, California

Alicia Mata, BS
Corinthian Colleges, Inc.
Santa Ana, California

Maureen Messier, AS, BA
Branford Hall Career Institute
Southington, Connecticut

Kathy Mooso, CMA
Idaho State University
Pocatello, Idaho

Lisa Nagle, BSEd, CMA
Augusta Technical College
Augusta, Georgia

Cora Newcomb
Technical College of the Lowcountry
Beaufort, South Carolina

Cheryl Startzell, MA, BS, AAS
San Antonio College
San Antonio, Texas

Kathy Steinberg, RN, BSN
Midwest Technical Institute
Lincoln, Illinois

Nina Thierer, BS
Ivy Tech Community College
Fort Wayne, Indiana

Stacey Wilson, BS, MT/PBT, CMA
Cabarrus College of Health Sciences
Concord, North Carolina

CONTENTS

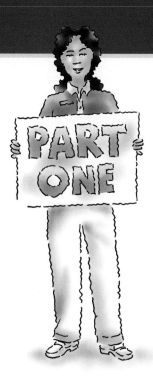

General Skills

Chapter 1
**COMMUNICATIONS SKILLS
FOR MEDICAL ASSISTANTS**

Chapter 2
**LAW AND ETHICS
FOR MEDICAL ASSISTANTS**

Chapter 3
OPERATIONAL FUNCTIONS

COMMUNICATIONS SKILLS FOR MEDICAL ASSISTANTS

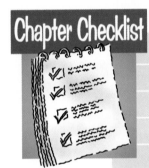

Chapter Checklist

- Recognize and respond to verbal communications
- Identify and describe six interviewing skills
- Recognize and respond to nonverbal communications
- Describe the skill of active listening
- List special techniques to use when talking to children and patients who are impaired or emotionally upset
- Summarize how to act professionally in your communications with patients and with other health care providers
- Identify community resources
- Explain why having a professional image in the office is important
- List the duties of a medical office receptionist
- Explain general office policies
- Demonstrate telephone techniques
- Identify the common types of incoming calls and explain how to handle each type
- Describe how to triage incoming calls
- Explain how to identify and handle calls that involve medical emergencies

- Respond to and initiate written communications

- List six key guidelines for medical writing

- Summarize how to write a business letter

- Name the ways written materials can be sent and explain how each method is used

- Describe the process for handling incoming mail

Communication is the sending and receiving of information. As a medical assistant, you will need good communication skills. You'll have to share information accurately with patients, physicians, and other health care workers. In this chapter, you'll learn about the various factors that can affect the accurate exchange of messages. You'll also learn techniques for communicating effectively in writing, over the telephone, and face-to-face in the medical office.

Communications Basics

Most information is communicated in messages. When we hear the word *message,* we probably think of voice mail or e-mail. These are just two kinds of messages. Messages may be spoken or written or they make take some other form. When dealing with patients, physicians, and coworkers, you must be able to receive and understand the messages they are sending. You also must be able to respond to those messages appropriately. You have to know what information to share and when and how to provide it.

Most likely, you'll be the first person a patient meets in the office. Your attitude and communication skills will set the tone for the rest of the patient's experience.

COMMUNICATION FLOW

Communication requires three things:

- a message
- a person to send the message
- a person to receive the message

In a conversation, people swing back and forth between the roles of sender and receiver. The receiver seeks **clarification** (understanding) of the message by sending a response called **feedback.**

As a medical assistant, one of your duties will be to communicate with patients. Good communication requires the following skills:

> Much of your communication will be conversations with patients about office policies, procedures, and patient care.

- *Clarifying.* State your message in a clear and direct way. For example, you can say, "I'm going to draw some blood now because the doctor would like to check your cholesterol level."

- *Validating.* Make sure your message answers the patient's questions or concerns. What if the patient asks if it is going to hurt? You might say, "You will feel a pinch when I insert the needle. I'll let you know when I'm going to do that."

- *Adapting.* Keep the patient's level of understanding in mind when stating a message. What if the patient asks if this is a routine test? You can answer, "Yes. This blood test is just part of a routine physical exam."

- *Questioning.* Ask the patient for feedback to be sure the message he received is the message you intended to send. For example, after you have drawn the blood, check in with the patient to be sure he doesn't have any questions. "We will contact you with the results of your cholesterol level. Do you have any further questions that I can answer?"

TYPES OF COMMUNICATION

The most common way of sending messages is by verbal communication. This form of communication uses language—words that are spoken or written. But not all messages involve the use of words. For example, you can often tell how a person feels about something by the expression on her face. Nonverbal communication is the sending and receiving of messages without using words.

Verbal Communication

Most of your communications as a medical assistant will be verbal communication. Much of that will involve oral communication—verbal communication that uses spoken words.

You'll need good oral communication skills to carry out many of your duties. You'll need to make appointments and referrals. You'll also educate patients about their conditions. And, of course, you'll be sharing information with the physician. These communication guidelines will help:

- Speak in a polite manner. A pleasant way of speaking is one sign of a professional.
- Use proper English. Bad grammar and slang expressions will give you an unprofessional image.
- Don't talk down to patients.
- Avoid using medical terms a patient might not know.

Other kinds of oral communication can change the meaning of spoken messages. Two examples of nonverbal "speech" are paralanguage and nonlanguage sounds.

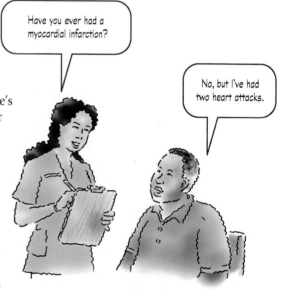

- *Paralanguage* includes a voice's tone, volume, and pitch. For example, someone who shouts, "I'm not angry!" at the top of his voice is sending a different message than a person who says the same thing in a quiet tone.
- *Nonlanguage sounds* include sighs, sobs, laughs, grunts, and so on. Such sounds can give spoken words very different meanings. For example, someone who says, "Everything is fine!" while sobbing is sending a message that he may not feel fine at all.

Knowing how to interpret paralanguage and nonlanguage sounds can help you plan your responses to the patient.

Written Communications. Using language to send written messages is another type of verbal communication. The ability to write clearly and accurately is another communication skill that is important in health care work. You'll read more about this skill later in this chapter.

After treatment, a patient usually receives oral instructions first. You or the physician will explain key areas of concern.

Closer Look

COMMUNICATING INSTRUCTIONS

If either oral or written instructions are unclear, the patient may not act correctly. This can slow or prevent the patient's recovery. The patient might even have to be admitted to the hospital. Here are some tips for communicating instructions.

- "Return to the office if you don't feel better" is an unclear instruction. It provides the patient with no details. Clearer instructions would say, "If your fever and sore throat are not better in 24 hours, call the office to schedule another visit."

- As a medical assistant, you are responsible for asking questions to make sure the patient clearly understands the information. A good question to ask about these instructions would be, "Do you need a card with the office's number in case you still have a fever and sore throat in 24 hours?"

Then the patient is generally given written instructions to take home. It's important that instructions are detailed and clear.

Nonverbal Communication

Nonverbal communication—sending messages without using words—is sometimes called *body language*. Body language includes several types of behavior, such as **kinesics, proxemics,** and touch.

Nonverbal communication can show more accurately a person's true feelings and attitude than verbal communication can. You must read people's nonverbal clues in addition to what they tell you.

Kinesics. Kinesics is the study of body movements. These include facial expressions, gestures, and eye movements. A patient's face can show inner feelings—such as anger

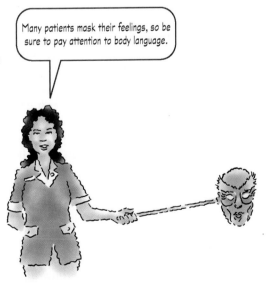

Many patients mask their feelings, so be sure to pay attention to body language.

or fear—that conversation may not reveal. The eyes can hint at what a person may be thinking or feeling. For example, a patient whose eyes wander while you are talking may be impatient or disinterested. Or he may not understand what you're saying.

Proxemics. Proxemics refers to a person's "comfort zone" and how she reacts to others in the space around her. People think of the area immediately around them as "personal space." Many people prefer that this space not be invaded by strangers. For most Americans, personal space extends out about three feet from their bodies.

First, I'm going to take your temperature, and then I'll get your blood pressure.

To provide care to patients, you must enter their personal space. Some people get very uncomfortable when their space is invaded. Therefore, it is important that you approach patients in a professional manner. You should explain clearly what you plan to do. Your explanation will make patients less anxious about what is going to happen.

Touch. For some patients, a kind, gentle touch can provide emotional support. But for other people, being touched by a stranger is a negative experience. It can make them very uncomfortable.

My Space

Before comforting a patient by touching, look for clues in the person's expressions and behavior that a touch would be accepted. Some people have negative feelings about being touched in a medical setting. Often, this is because they connect being touched with something unpleasant, such as getting an injection. Such feelings can be overcome, however. One way is to offer a comforting touch at times when nothing unpleasant or painful is about to follow.

ACTIVE LISTENING

Active listening helps you understand the messages the patient is sending. If you do not receive and interpret a patient's messages correctly, you will not be able to provide the best care.

Active listening is a skill that must be developed. You become an active listener by following these practices:

- Give your full attention to the person who is speaking.

- Keep interruptions to a minimum.

- Pay attention to the speaker's paralanguage, body language, and other clues, in addition to what she is saying.

Following the Hands On procedure on page 55, on recognizing and using nonverbal clues, will also help you be a better active listener.

Suppose a patient is wringing his hands as he tells you that everything is fine. This could be a nonverbal message that is in conflict with his verbal one.

INTERVIEWING PATIENTS

As a medical assistant, it's likely that one of your duties will be taking information from new patients. You also may be updating information on existing patients. You'll perform either duty by interviewing the patient. You'll need to ask certain questions and interpret the patient's responses.

New patient interviews cover several topics. They include the patient's medical and family history, a brief review of body systems, and the patient's social history and medications. The key subjects in each area are listed in the table.

An interview of a patient who has seen the physician before—called an **established patient**—is quite different. You should take these steps when interviewing an established patient.

1. Review the patient's chart for information about her health problems.

2. Make a list of questions to ask the patient to update health information about current medical problems and any changes in health.

3. Confirm with the patient that she is still on the medications and treatments listed on the chart.

4. Ask about any allergies.

Effective interviews with new and established patients require good communication skills. Show professionalism during the interview. Begin by introducing yourself. Listen actively. Ask the appropriate questions and carefully record answers. Finally, always conduct the interview in a private area. The Hands On section on page 56 offers more tips that will make you a better interviewer, as well as a better communicator overall.

Key Subjects in a New Patient Interview

Key Subjects	What You Need to Know
Medical History	Any hospitalizations and dates
	Any surgeries and dates
	Any chronic problems
Female Patients	Any pregnancies and complications
	Any miscarriages, stillbirths, or abortions
Family History	Age and health of parents (if deceased, cause and age at death)
	Age and health of brothers and sisters
	Any genetic problems in family
Body System Review	General questions about all body systems: cardiovascular, pulmonary, integumentary, musculoskeletal, sensory, neurological, gastrointestinal, immune, endocrine, urological, and reproductive
Social History	Alcohol use
	Tobacco use
	Any drug use
	Hobbies
	Education
	Employment
Medications	Any prescription medicines (when taken and how much)
	Any over-the-counter medicines (when taken and how much)
	Any vitamins and herbal supplements

PATIENT EDUCATION

As a medical assistant, you'll need good communication skills to teach patients about their medical conditions. Teaching can involve something as simple as explaining how often a patient should take a medication.

The communication skills involved in patient teaching include skills for active listening and interviewing. Follow these guidelines to provide effective patient education:

- Find a quiet room away from the main office flow, if possible.

- Have useful handouts or information sheets available.

- Allow enough teaching time so you're not rushed.

- Give information in a clear, organized, and to-the-point manner.

- Follow the oral teaching with written instructions.

- Allow the patient time to review the written instructions.

- Encourage the patient to ask questions.

- Ask questions in a way that will help you know whether or not the patient understands the instruction.

- Invite the patient to call the office if any other questions come to mind.

Stay aware of current medical issues, discoveries, and trends, as well as useful community services that are available in your area. This knowledge will make you an even better patient educator. The Hands On procedure on page 57 will guide you in identifying and using community resources to help meet patients' needs.

CHALLENGES TO GOOD COMMUNICATION

Sometimes, no matter how hard you try, people may not receive your message accurately. This is especially true if you use slang and clichés. A cliché is an expression that has lost its original meaning.

The problem is that the patient may not understand the meaning of the cliché. This is especially likely if the patient's native language is not English. Patients who are not in your general age group also may not understand your clichés. You should avoid the use of slang terms for the same reason.

There are some other common reasons why patients may misunderstand your message.

- *You used medical terms.* Keep in mind that most patients will not understand many medical terms and abbreviations. If you use such terms in speaking to patients, be sure they understand what the terms mean.

- *The patient was distracted.* A common cause of distraction is pain. For example, teaching a patient how to use crutches is much more difficult if his ankle or knee still hurts. He will be concentrating on the pain, not on what you are saying. The same is true of patients who have just received good news. Their focus will be on calling family members and not on your conversation.

- *Environmental factors interfered.* Noise or interruptions can distort messages. For example, staff lounges or break rooms can be noisy. Keep the doors to these areas closed. Also, workers should not be vacuuming or emptying trash while patients are present.

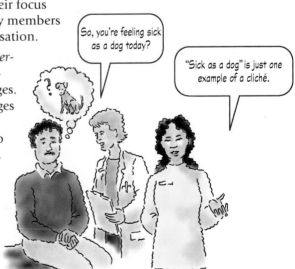

So, you're feeling sick as a dog today?

"Sick as a dog" is just one example of a cliché.

Cultural Differences

In your medical assisting career, you'll come into

contact with people from many backgrounds and cultures. Each person's culture shapes his values and beliefs. A person's background often influences the way that person views other people and situations. Understanding these differences can help you give each patient the best care.

Patients from some cultures may be offended by the personal questions asked when their medical history is taken. They may view such questions as an invasion of their privacy. In such cases, the physician may need to get involved to lessen the patient's concerns.

It might seem harmless to casually touch a patient on the arm when talking to him. Many people, however, don't like to be touched—especially by someone they don't know. There are also cultural differences that you must consider. For example, in Asian cultures, it is not appropriate to touch a person's head. If this comes up during a medical procedure, you should explain yourself and make sure the patient is comfortable.

As we discussed earlier, personal space also can be an issue. Americans feel comfortable with about three feet of personal space, although this varies in different cultures. Look for non-verbal clues that show a patient's comfort level before you move in for an exam.

Be sensitive to these differences when you interact with patients. This reduces misunderstandings and helps avoid offending patients.

Closer Look   SEEING EYE-TO-EYE

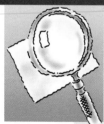

Looking people directly in the eyes is viewed differently in some cultures. In the United States, good eye contact usually makes a person seem honest and concerned. Other cultures, however, feel differently about eye contact.

- In some cultures, including Asian and Native American cultures, direct eye contact is viewed as disrespectful. It may even seem sexually suggestive or aggressive.

- In other cultures, including Latino cultures, avoiding eye contact or casting the eyes downward is a sign of respect.

Bias and Stereotyping

As a medical assistant, you'll meet people of differing ages, races, and sexual orientations. Your values sometimes may differ greatly from a patient's values. But you should never let your values or your **bias** (opinions about something) affect your dealings with patients. To treat them differently because of their backgrounds, cultures, or personal values is **discrimination.**

Stereotyping is holding an opinion about all members of a group based on oversimplified views about some of its members. Stereotyping is a form of **prejudice.**

Bias, discrimination, stereotyping, and prejudice have no place in health care. These damaging views don't allow for patients' individual differences. They also prevent everyone from receiving quality care on an equal basis.

As a health care professional, you have a duty to treat all people fairly and equally. The following practices will help you do this:

- Avoid letting stereotypes shape your opinions.
- Don't make value judgments about people.
- Have a professional attitude and manner.
- Guard against discrimination in your practices.

By doing these things, you send patients the message that you accept human differences. This will give them confidence that you provide quality care to all who seek it.

> All patients must be treated fairly, respectfully, and with dignity, regardless of their cultural, social, or personal values.

Language Barriers

The best communication takes place when language is used. But some people cannot speak or understand enough English for effective communication. You may need to use an interpreter in such cases. Someone on the office staff also might be able to help. In either case, be sure the interpreter accurately understands what you are saying.

It may seem logical to use an English-speaking member of the patient's family as an interpreter. However, this should only be a last resort. Family members might feel uncomfortable sharing bad news or information of a sensitive nature.

When choosing an interpreter, try to find someone of the same gender as the patient. Some cultures ban members of the opposite gender—even family members— from discussing personal issues about the body.

If a good interpreter is not available, a phrase book of common medical questions may be helpful. These books also list possible answers to each question. You might also keep a book of pictures or photos on hand to help in these situations. There are also toll-free numbers that provide interpreters that could help in an emergency.

> If your area has a large number of people who speak a certain language, your office should have a medical phrase book for that language.

Other Communication Challenges

Many situations present special challenges for communication. Some patients may have sight or hearing problems. Patients may be young children or they may be too ill or medicated to understand. Other patients may have limited understanding due to mental or emotional conditions. Patients who are frightened or anxious may require even more special attention.

In each case, you need to evaluate the situation and the patient's ability to understand. Many times, a family member will be present who can help you. Make sure to obtain all needed information, whether that involves the patient or the family member. But never completely ignore the patient. Patients should feel they are part of the exchange, even when it requires the help of others.

Hearing-Impaired Patients. Hearing impairments can range from partial hearing loss to complete hearing loss. Patients with complete hearing loss are usually able to communicate with sign language, interpreters, or other tools. Those with partial hearing loss can be a bigger challenge. This condition is common among elderly people, who may be unwilling to accept their reduced ability to hear.

Communicating with all hearing-impaired patients requires sensitivity and patience. These suggestions may help:

- Touch the patient gently to gain her attention.
- Talk directly in front of the patient, face to face. Don't place yourself at an angle to the patient or talk with your back turned.
- Make sure you are near a bright light, so that your face is illuminated.

Closer Look

COMMUNICATING WITH NON–ENGLISH-SPEAKING PATIENTS

Here are some suggestions and guidelines for talking with patients who do not speak English well:

- Speak slowly. Use simple sentences and phrases that require simple answers. The patient may understand some simple English.
- Avoid using slang. It may not translate well.
- Do not shout. Raising your voice will not increase the patient's understanding.
- Use gestures as needed. Gestures tend to be widely understood.
- Speak directly to the patient if you're using an interpreter. This will allow you to read each other's facial expressions.
- Avoid distractions and provide a relaxed, quiet interview space.
- Use pictures and other communication aids if necessary.
- Learn some basic phrases of the most common language used in your area. Patients will appreciate your effort

---

- Use short sentences with short words. Speak clearly and with force. Don't exaggerate your facial movements.
- Don't shout. In most cases, shouting doesn't help. In fact, it can distort what is heard.
- Lower the pitch of your voice. People with some kinds of partial hearing loss cannot hear high-pitched sounds.
- Use notepads and demonstrations as needed. Pictograms—flash cards that show basic medical terms—can be helpful.
- Eliminate all distractions. Nearby noises can confuse patients with partial hearing loss.

Sight-Impaired Patients. Sight impairments range from complete blindness to blurred vision. Patients who can't see lose information others gain from nonverbal communication.

Here are some ideas for communicating with sight-impaired patients:

- Identify yourself by name each time the patient comes into the office.

- Speak in a normal tone without raising your voice. The patient is not hearing impaired.
- At all times, let the patient know exactly what you'll be doing. Alert the patient before touching him or her.
- Offer the patient your arm and escort him to the examining or interview room.
- Have the patient touch the examining table, counter, chair, etc., to help him gain a mental image of the room.
- Explain the sounds of any machines to be used in the examination or procedure and what each machine does.
- Tell the patient when you are leaving the room and knock before entering.

Speech Impairments. Speech impairments can come from a number of medical conditions. One common condition is stroke. Oral surgery and cancer of the tongue or voice box also can affect a patient's ability to communicate, as can stuttering.

These suggestions will help you communicate with a patient who has a speech impairment:

- Allow such patients time to gather their thoughts.
- Allow plenty of time for them to communicate.
- Don't rush conversations.
- Be aware of your own facial expressions.
- Offer a notepad to write questions.

Mental Health Conditions. Many mental disorders can damage a patient's ability to communicate. These disorders present a wide range of challenges. Some illnesses can cause the patient to have uncontrolled outbursts. Others can keep the patient from communicating at all. Some patients may hear voices that tell them what to say.

Communicating with patients who have moderate to severe mental disorders requires special training and practice. But many patients with mental illnesses will not offer such challenges. Most mental illnesses can be controlled with medication and other treatments.

Use these methods when communicating with patients who have mental illnesses:

- Tell the patient what to expect and when things will happen.
- Keep conversations professional and focused.
- Don't force or demand answers from patients who will not speak.

- Don't agree with a patient who asks if you are hearing voices or seeing objects that are not there.
- Try to help return a patient to reality if appropriate.

If you feel unsafe with the patient, speak to your supervisor or the physician about your concerns.

> Remember that it's not your job to recommend treatment or counseling for patients with substance abuse problems.

Substance Abuse. It also can be difficult to communicate with patients who have histories of substance abuse, alcoholism, or other addictions. If they are withdrawing from addiction, they may be very upset and aggressive. When dealing with such patients, keep the following points in mind:

- Identify the reason for their visit and follow your regular assessment duties.
- Keep your communication professional.
- Avoid making any judgments about them.
- Speak in a calm voice.

Angry or Distressed Patients. Illness, long waiting times, and financial issues are among the things that can make some patients angry or upset. The key to communicating with such patients is to keep the problem from getting worse. Tell patients about waiting times, billing and insurance practices, and office policies that might make them upset.

It's common for patients to get upset when they hear bad news about their health. Most patients take such news in a calm manner. But it's important to offer assistance as needed.

Provide written instructions for the patient to read later. They should include information of the diagnosis, causes of the illness, treatment choices, and phone numbers to call for more information.

Most importantly, you don't want to get defensive. Here are some suggestions to help you communicate with an angry or distressed patient:

- Be supportive.
- Be open and honest.
- Don't give the patient false reassurances.
- Don't make light of the patient's problem or concern.
- Avoid using humor and sarcasm.
- Ensure your own safety if the patient becomes aggressive or threatening.
- Speak in a low, calm voice.

Children. Children's levels of understanding vary greatly. Communication must be adjusted to each child's needs. The following general suggestions will help you.

- Children respond to eye contact on their level. Raise them to your height, or, better yet, lower yourself to theirs.
- Keep your voice low-pitched and gentle.
- If you think the child doesn't understand a question, ask it in a different way.
- Keep your movements slow and visible. Tell children when you need to touch them.
- Allow a child to express fear, to cry, and so on.
- Be prepared for the child to return to an earlier stage of development during an illness. For example, a child may go back to thumb sucking for comfort during times of stress.
- If a child doesn't want to talk, use play to ask your question and get the child's cooperation.

There are also hints for communicating effectively with adolescents. Here are some tips.

- Many adolescents resent authority. Some teenagers may not want a parent in the room during the interview. Assess the situation before including the parent.
- Never show shock or judgment when dealing with adolescents. Doing so will immediately close communication.

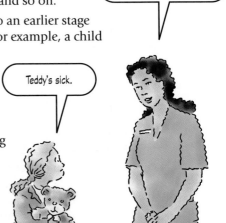

I'm sorry to hear that. And how do you feel?

Teddy's sick.

TALKING THROUGH THE STEPS

When dealing with children, you want to clearly explain exactly what you will be doing. You should tell them about every step in a procedure so that there are no surprises.

Suppose you are going to take a child's temperature using a tympanic thermometer. You can't just say, "I'm going to take your temperature." Instead, you want to explain the steps in the process.

- First, you might say, "Now I am going to take your temperature. Are you ready?"
- Next, before you place the probe into the ear, you can say, "I'm going to put this small part right inside of your ear. Don't worry, it's not going to hurt."
- Then, you might say, "Could you hold still for me just until I say it's okay to move?"
- Finally, when you finish, you want to praise the child for doing a great job.

Grieving Patients. At times, you'll encounter patients or family members who are dealing with **grief,** or great sadness. Grieving starts when a person suffers an important loss. This might be the death of a loved one, the end of a relationship, the loss of a job, or the loss of good health or a body part.

Grieving is a complex process that usually takes place in the following stages.

1. denial
2. anger
3. bargaining
4. depression
5. acceptance

The stages don't have to occur in this order. Some people might experience the stages in a different order. Others might skip stages in the process. Every person is different.

Each stage in the process can produce certain emotions and behaviors. In the anger stage, a patient may blame the physician or the care he received at the medical office. The depression stage can lead to unusual quietness, isolation, and increased crying. Acceptance is the last stage. The patient may say, "I understand that I have a terminal disease and that I am going to die." A **terminal disease** is a fatal illness that is in its final stages.

The stages of grieving can spread over many months. Each person grieves at his own pace and in his own way. There's no set time period and no right way to grieve. Some grieving patients may want to talk about their feelings. Patients with a terminal disease might want to discuss their fears of dying. They may express concern for loved ones they will leave behind.

Support grieving patients in the following ways:

- Give grieving patients the time to express themselves. Practice active listening.

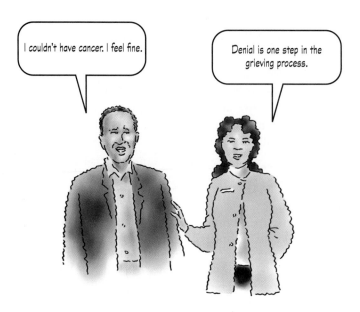

- Use touch to show your understanding if the situation is appropriate.
- Provide education for patients if some of their concerns are because of a lack of understanding about their condition.
- Be familiar with local resources such as grief or other counseling services and hospice care. Your awareness allows you to suggest such services when they are needed.

PROFESSIONAL DISTANCE

How people act toward each other is determined by their relationships. For instance, you treat a friend differently than you would a stranger. Your dealings with patients must be at a level that allows you to carry out your duties effectively. You must not let personal relationships affect how you do that.

It's easy to get attached to patients, especially elderly patients who may be lonely. But getting personally involved with patients is not a good idea. It can damage your ability to make objective decisions about these patients and their needs. Here are some tips.

- Don't offer to drive patients to appointments, pick up prescriptions, or do their grocery shopping. Keep your professional distance. This helps you stay objective. It also makes the care you deliver more professional and effective.

Closer Look  DEALING WITH DEATH AND DYING

It's normal to feel sad when a patient is dying or passes away. But it's important that your communication does not focus on sympathy. Instead, you should focus on empathy. The difference is this—sympathy can be described as feeling *for* someone, but empathy is feeling *with* someone. In health care, that means trying to understand what patients are feeling so you can help them. Having sympathy or pity for a patient could cause you to become personally involved in the patient's situation. That would be a highly unprofessional thing to do.

- Another way of keeping a professional distance is to avoid talking to patients about yourself. Avoid any topics, such as family or financial problems, that could shift your relationship with a patient to a more personal level.

> Empathy can help you recognize a patient's fear and discomfort so you can do everything possible to provide support.

Professional Communications

Good communication with your coworkers is just as important as good communication with your patients.

Communicating with Coworkers

Conversations with coworkers must be appropriate and professional throughout the workday. Discussions that aren't related to work should be limited to break times. It's not appropriate to discuss TV shows, family problems, and so on in front of patients. Loud talking, whispering, and a lot of laughing also create an unprofessional environment.

Communicating with Physicians

Physicians depend on medical assistants for information they need to provide quality patient care. This communication always must be professional. Follow these guidelines when talking with a physician:

- Always call the physician *doctor* unless she tells you otherwise.
- Never call the physician by her first name in front of a patient.

Closer Look   PROPER FORMS OF ADDRESS

How you address patients sends them clues about your attitude and how you will provide care.

- A proper form of address, such as *Mrs. Smith* or *Mr. Jones,* shows respect and sets a professional tone.

- Nicknames, such as *sweetie, honey,* and *kiddo* aren't appropriate in a medical setting. They can offend patients' dignity. Using nicknames also puts communication on a personal level instead of a professional one.

- Avoid identifying patients by their medical condition, such as "the broken arm in the waiting room." Patients who come to a medical office often feel anxious. This can make them very sensitive to things they see and hear. Using medical conditions instead of names can be insulting to many patients. It sends the message that staff members see them as nothing more than an illness.

- Avoid using slang in place of proper medical terms. For example, say *urine* instead of *pee.* If you're unsure of the correct term, explain the condition instead. That's better than using a term that might be incorrect.

- Speak confidently to earn the physician's trust and respect.

- Be honest if you don't know something. It's better to say, "I'm not sure what to do with this specimen," than to do something and make a mistake.

Communicating with Other Offices

Physicians sometimes send patients to other offices for special treatments, tests, or services. This action is called a **referral.** Physicians often depend on their medical assistants to make the arrangements. Keep these key points in mind when you make a referral:

- The patient's privacy always comes first. Make sure that you give no more medical information about the patient than the other office needs.

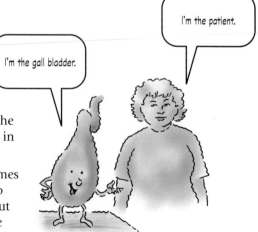

Closer Look | PROTECTING PATIENTS' PRIVACY

Information about patients is confidential. This means it must be kept private. To help keep patient information from being revealed accidentally, practice these behaviors in the office each and every day:

- Be careful not to speak too loudly.
- When calling coworkers over an intercom, do not reveal the patient's name or other information. For example, don't say, "Bob Smith is on the phone. He wants to know if his blood test results are back." Instead, just say, "There's a patient on line 1."
- Don't discuss patients in cafeterias, elevators, parking lots, or other public places. A patient's friends or relatives might overhear you.
- Before going home, destroy any slips of paper in your pockets that have notes about patients on them.
- If there is a window between the reception desk and the waiting area, keep it closed when not speaking to visitors.

- Follow all legal requirements for giving the information to the new office.
- Be careful when using fax machines, e-mail, and other electronic devices. Make sure the intended receiver is the one who gets the information.
- Provide only facts. Don't relay suspicions or assumptions about the patient.
- Don't make judgments about the information or the patient when communicating with the other office.
- Make sure the other office received the information and that it can do the referral.

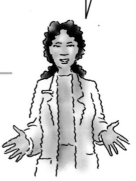

You must respect a patient's privacy when giving patient information to other health care providers.

Attitude, Appearance, and Impression

As a medical assistant, you'll be the patient's main contact with the physician. In some cases, a patient may spend more time with you than with the physician. You're also likely to be the first office professional the patient meets. If your duties include working at the reception desk or answering the phone, this will always be true.

Your attitude and appearance send messages to patients as much as your verbal and nonverbal communications do. First impressions are lasting ones. The way you look and the way you interact with the patient will set the tone for the visit. It will influence how the patient views the office and the quality of care it provides.

The importance of presenting yourself to patients as a qualified and caring professional cannot be overemphasized.

> Remember, you have only ONE chance to make a good first impression on patients.

- A positive view of the office helps create a good physician-patient relationship.
- Patients who feel positive about their experience are more likely to follow their treatment plan.
- Patients with a negative view of the office may choose to find another physician.
- Loss of patients will cause a loss of income for the office. (A medical office is like any other business. It will not keep operating if does not make money.)

Courtesy and Diplomacy

Success as a medical assistant requires courtesy and diplomacy. Courtesy is politeness and good manners. Diplomacy is the art of dealing with people in difficult situations without offending them. Both skills are basic to good human relations.

Here are just a few ways to show courtesy and respect to coworkers.

- Ask permission before borrowing supplies or using someone else's desk.
- Always knock before entering a room, even if the door is open.
- Refer to physicians by their title and last name, unless they tell you otherwise.

Every day, you will deal with many different people in different circumstances. You have to remain positive and professional, even at difficult times.

Use diplomacy in touchy situations. For example, patients may want to know what's wrong with other patients. Family members may want to know what the physician told the patient. You must politely refuse to give out such information. It is confidential.

Pain, worry, and waiting can make a patient angry or un-reasonable. You must use self-control and continue to act professionally. Never argue with a patient. Try to calm the patient and show your desire to help. Finally, any situation that you can't handle should be referred to the physician or office manager.

> By showing understanding, interest, and concern, you tell a patient that he is important and that you care.

The Importance of Attitude

Your attitude is the way you feel about something. It can be either positive or negative. How you feel influences how you act. You transfer your attitude to others through your behavior. You have the power to influence a patient's attitude and behavior.

As a medical assistant, you must be able to transfer a positive attitude to patients. This requires that you view every person as someone who is worthy of care and respect. Ask yourself: "If I were in this patient's situation, how would I want to be treated?" Your positive attitude toward a patient will influence her own attitude and behavior. In this way, your actions can lead to a more positive response from the patient.

GOOD ATTITUDE IN ACTION

Suppose you are working at the reception desk one day during flu season. A patient arrives and sees other patients in the waiting room ahead of him. He grumbles about being on time for his appointment but still having to wait. Which of these responses shows the patient a positive attitude?

- "I know you feel terrible, Mr. Smith, but so does everyone else in the waiting room. It's the flu season. Just have a seat, and the doctor will see you shortly."

- "I'm sorry you feel so bad, Mr. Smith. Do you feel well enough to sit in the waiting room for about ten minutes? The doctor should be ready to see you by then."

The second message tells the patient that you care about how he feels. It also reassures him that he will see the physician soon. The attitude sent in the first message was that Mr. Smith was just one more sick patient. Mr. Smith's attitude will probably be improved by receiving the second message. Therefore; he will probably respond better to the second message than to the first one.

The Importance of Appearance

Your appearance is another factor that will influence how a patient views the medical office. Good health and good grooming present a positive image to the patient.

One way you can affect your appearance is by taking good care of yourself. Taking "good care" of yourself means:

- eating the "right" foods (having a balanced diet)
- exercising regularly (even walking will help)
- getting enough sleep (but not at work, of course)

These tips will help not only your appearance, but also your performance. If you are tired or sluggish, you cannot provide good patient care.

Personal Hygiene. Pay special attention to personal hygiene. People who are ill are often very sensitive to odors. Even smells that are normally pleasant can be distressing to them. A daily shower or bath is important, followed by an unscented deodorant. Do not wear perfume, cologne, or scented lotions or hair spray. Good oral hygiene is also important. During the day, avoid foods that may produce an offensive odor, such as garlic or onions.

Grooming. Keep your hair clean and styled. Fingernails must be clean and trimmed. If you wear nail polish, use only clear or neutral polish. Vivid colors are not appropriate for a medical office. Long nails also are not appropriate. If you wear makeup, keep it natural and apply it lightly.

Dress. Most offices have a dress code. Here are some general guidelines.

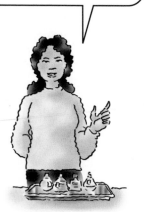

Save your favorite perfume for the weekends, not the workplace.

- Whether you wear a uniform or not, your clothes should be clean and pressed. Wrinkles, stains, missing buttons, and tears do not create a professional image.
- Your shoes should always be clean and polished.
- Women's stockings should be neutral in color and free of runs and holes.
- Women's jewelry should be plain and simple. Large rings, long chains, dangling earrings, and showy bracelets are not appropriate for the medical office. Multiple bracelets also are not appropriate jewelry for a medical setting.
- If you have pierced ears, many offices require that you wear only small stud earrings. In some offices, you can

Closer Look

GUIDELINES FOR NAILS

The Centers for Disease Control (CDC) is a U.S. government agency. It's part of the Department of Health and Human Services. The CDC has issued guidelines for the fingernails of health care workers. These guidelines call for natural nail tips to be less than a quarter-inch long.

The CDC also strongly discourages health care providers from wearing artificial nails. Artificial nails increase the chance an infection could be passed between the provider and a patient. According to CDC guidelines, any health care providers who work with high-risk patients must not wear artificial nails.

only wear one pair of earrings and you must remove any facial piercings.

- If you have any tattoos, don't be surprised if you're asked to cover them up while at work. This is standard practice for many offices.

The Medical Assistant as Receptionist

Medical offices often hire a nonmedical person to serve as receptionists. The receptionist is the employee who greets patients and alerts the appropriate staff members when patients arrive. In many offices, the receptionist also answers the telephone. If you work in this kind of office, your duties may include filling in for the receptionist while he is at lunch or on break.

In some offices, you may work as a receptionist all or most of the time. These offices prefer to have a medically trained person in this role. But whichever type of office you are in, you need to know and be able to perform the duties of a receptionist.

BEFORE THE OFFICE OPENS

A receptionist's duties start before the first patient arrives. Her first duties might include:

- unlocking the door and turning on the lights
- turning off an alarm, if necessary

Closer Look   THE ANSWERING SERVICE

Answering services take calls from patients and others when the office is closed. If a call is urgent, the answering service will contact the physician or the physician's nurse practitioner, usually by pager. The physician or nurse practitioner will then return the patient's call. Non-emergency calls are held by the service until the office opens the next day.

- turning on computers, printers, copiers, and other electronic equipment
- checking that the examination rooms have been cleaned and are stocked with needed supplies
- checking that the reception room, bathrooms, and other public spaces are clean
- checking for any messages on the answering machine or voice mail, on the fax machine, in e-mail, or left with the answering service overnight
- checking that the thermostat is set to a comfortable temperature

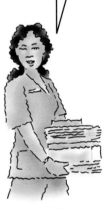

Restock your desk with the supplies and forms you need before the first patients arrive.

Preparing the Charts

One of your most important duties is to gather the charts of all patients who will be seen during the day.

Put the charts in order of the patients' appointments. Preparing the day's charts also includes the following tasks:

- Review each chart. Make sure it is complete and updated.
- Check that blank progress notes are in the chart for the physician to write his notes.
- If this is the patient's first visit, make up a new chart. Include with the chart any forms new patients must fill out. You should also include any medical records from another office.

Most offices pull the charts the day before so they are ready in the morning. If you wait until the morning, there might not be time to locate any paperwork missing from the files.

The prepared charts for the day are usually kept at the reception desk. The receptionist then gives each chart to the physician or the clinical assistant when the patient arrives.

WHILE THE OFFICE IS OPEN

During the medical office's business day, your main responsibilities as receptionist will include:

- welcoming patients and visitors
- registering and orienting patients
- managing the reception area

Welcoming Patients and Visitors

Try to greet all patients in person and by name, if possible. A smile and cheerful greeting make the patient feel welcome. This helps create a positive image of the office for the patient. Try to recall something personal about the patient. Ask about a hobby or pet.

Sometimes, a patient will arrive while you are away from your desk. Check the reception area for new arrivals when you return. Many offices have a bell or chime on the door. Some have a sign asking patients to check in with the receptionist.

Registering and Orienting Patients

Patients who are new to the office will have to fill out a registration form, or a patient information sheet. They also must sign a privacy notice that's required by federal law.

The registration form asks the patient to provide some basic information:

- the patient's name, address, phone number, and social security number
- the name, address, and phone number of the patient's insurance company, or whoever is responsible for paying the bill
- the name and address of the patient's employer
- the patient's marital status and spouse's name, if appropriate
- the name of the person who referred the patient

Many information sheets also ask about the patient's health history. Sometimes, you will complete this part of the form while interviewing the patient. But most offices have the patient fill in this information. He can ask for your help if he has any questions.

The **Health Insurance Portability and Accountability Act of 1996 (HIPAA)** requires medical offices to inform patients how they handle patients' personal and health information. This notice must be given at the patient's first visit. By signing it, the patient agrees that he understands and accepts the office's privacy policies.

After the patient has completed this paperwork, briefly explain the office's general policies. The Hands On procedure on page 58 provides step-by-step guidelines for doing this. When it's the patient's turn to be seen, you may also be responsible for escorting the patient to the examination room.

Reception Area Management

Another important receptionist duty is managing the reception area. This area should provide safety and comfort for patients waiting to be seen by medical staff. It should be clean and uncluttered with plenty of room for walking. Check the reception area several times a day to make sure it is clean and tidy.

Managing Waiting Time. Patients expect to be seen at their appointment time. They've taken time from their schedules to see the physician. They don't want to be kept waiting.

Be sure to tell patients if the physician is behind schedule. If you expect the wait will be more than 30 minutes from their appointment time, offer patients some choices.

Long waiting times are among patients' greatest complaints.

- Ask the patient if he wants to reschedule her appointment for another day.
- Suggest that the patient leave the office and come back at a later time that day if she wishes.

You'll read more about scheduling appointments and on making adjustments in the schedule in Chapter 4.

The Reception Area and Contagious Diseases. It's important that patients in the reception area not be exposed to others with contagious diseases. This is a greater concern in some offices than in others. Family practice physicians and **pediatricians** (children's physicians) often treat highly contagious diseases. If you work for a pediatrician, you'll need to learn how to look at rashes and tell if they are contagious.

Managing patients with contagious diseases requires good communication with the clinical staff. They may know if one of the day's patients has a contagious disease. If so, they should alert you.

Many infectious diseases cannot by passed by routine contact, such as shaking hands, talking, or touching. Examples of such diseases are HIV and hepatitis. Some diseases however, are highly contagious, and patients who have them should not be left in the reception area.

If a patient has one of these conditions, she should not wait in the reception area with other patients. Patients with the following should be taken to an examination room at once:

- chickenpox
- conjunctivitis
- influenza
- measles and rubella
- meningitis (and suspected cases)
- mumps
- pertussis
- pneumonia (if patient is coughing)
- smallpox
- tuberculosis
- wounds (if open and draining)

Other patients may have impaired immune systems. For instance, medications they are taking may lower their resistance to infection. (Some treatments for cancer do this.) "Germs" that would be harmless to other people can be dangerous to such patients. To reduce their risk of exposure, they also should wait in an examination room. Every office should have guidelines for handling these patients.

Some pediatric offices have two waiting rooms—one for sick children and one for well children.

Patients with Disabilities

Federal law requires that all public places be available to people with disabilities. A medical reception area is a place that is open to the public. The "public" in this case includes patients and their families.

The Americans with Disabilities Act (ADA) sets requirements for buildings so that people with disabilities can use them. Some basic requirements that apply to medical offices appear in the table on page 32.

As a receptionist, you have no control over the structure of the office. But there are some things you can do to help make its public areas "friendly" to people with disabilities.

- Ask that all deliveries be left in a safe place. They shouldn't be left in the reception area or where they block doorways.
- Keep toys clear of pathways into and through the waiting room.
- Check that chairs aren't placed where they might block the movement of a wheelchair.

- Make sure doors are not blocked or propped open with objects.
- Check the restroom occasionally to make sure the entrance is open and not blocked.
- Limit stacks of papers on counters that might limit patients' access to you.

Summary of ADA Requirements for Public Buildings

Area	Requirements
Access	Route must be at least 36 inches wide.
	Route must be stable, firm, and have a no-slip surface.
Ramps	Ramps must be 36 inches wide.
	Railings must be 34–38 inches high.
	Ramps longer than 6 feet must have 2 railings.
	All public levels must have ramps and elevators.
Doors	Doors must be 32 inches wide.
	Door handles must be no higher than 48 inches.
	Handles must allow doors to be opened with a closed fist.
	Inside doors must open without using great force.
Restrooms	Restrooms must be identified by signs that can be read by touch.
	Doorway must be at least 32 inches wide.
	Doors (including stall doors), soap dispensers, hand dryers, and faucets must be able to be operated by a closed fist.
	A wheelchair stall is required; it must be at least 5 feet by 5 feet in size.
Other	Carpeting must be no more than a half-inch high.
	Emergency exit system must have flashing lights and sound signals.
	Tables and counters must be 28–34 inches high.
	Space for wheelchair seating must be available.

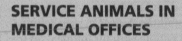

Ask the Professional   SERVICE ANIMALS IN MEDICAL OFFICES

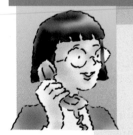

Q: *One of our new patients is blind. She arrived for her first appointment with her seeing-eye dog. I told her that we can't allow animals in the office and that one of us would help her while she was here. She had to reschedule her appointment because she had nowhere to leave her dog. She seemed a little upset. Did I do the right thing?*

A: The Americans with Disabilities Act (ADA) forbids businesses from banning service animals. A service animal is any animal that is trained to assist a person

Ask the Professional **SERVICE ANIMALS IN MEDICAL OFFICES (*continued*)**

with a disability. The law applies even if the patient's dog isn't officially licensed as a service animal. Besides seeing-eye dogs, service animals include those that alert hearing-impaired patients to sounds, pick up things for patients who have difficulty moving, and sense smells for seizure patients. They must not be separated from their owner and should be allowed to go with the patient to the examination room.

When a patient arrives with a service animal, it's a good idea to have him wait in an empty examining room. Some people in the general waiting room might be afraid of animals or children might try and play with them.

Telephone Techniques

The telephone is the main communication tool of the medical office. You must be able to create a positive image of the office when you answer the phone. This can be more difficult than in a face-to-face conversation.

In a phone conversation, nonverbal aids such as appearance and body language cannot help. For this reason, excellent verbal skills are needed to project a caring and professional attitude over the phone. It also helps to smile when you answer the phone. This may sound silly, but you will come across sounding cheerful and professional.

PHONE COURTESY

The tone and quality of your voice and speech shape the impression you send over the phone. Here are some guidelines for answering the phone in a way that is courteous and professional.

- Answer incoming calls promptly—by the second ring, if possible.
- Identify the office and yourself to the caller and offer assistance. This lets the caller know he has reached the correct number. For example, answer by saying, "Dr. Smith's office, Ms. Jones speaking. Can I help you?"

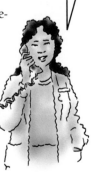

Answering calls promptly lets patients know they're important.

- Always speak politely, even if the call has interrupted your work. Do not allow your voice to show impatience or irritation.
- Never answer the phone and immediately put the caller on hold. Ask if the caller would mind holding. Courtesy requires that you wait for an answer. Also, you must find out if the call is an emergency before putting it on hold.

Running Smoothly — TRIAGING INCOMING CALLS

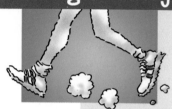

Your telephone has four incoming lines. This allows several patients to call at once. Suppose the following calls were on the lines at the same time:

- Line 1: The caller wants to make an appointment for her son, who has a 101.3° fever.
- Line 2: The caller wants to see the physician this afternoon. He's having chest pains.
- Line 3: The caller is upset because she's been disconnected three times. She has a question about her bill.
- Line 4: The caller needs a prescription refill.

You must **triage** *these calls. That means sort them into order of importance. Which call would you handle first? Which second? Which last?*

- Talk to the caller on line 2 first. Any possible life-threatening situation must have top priority. Follow your office policy on emergencies in handling this call. In some offices, you would transfer the call to a nurse, who would assess the situation. In others, you would advise the patient to call 911.
- Take caller 3 next. The longer she waits, the more upset she'll be. That will make her more difficult to please.
- Then make the appointment for caller 1, following your office policies on patient care issues.
- The caller on line 4 is last because he has the least urgent need.

One tip for triaging calls is to keep a notebook by the phone. You can use it to make notes about who is calling and why. This will help you remember the details and decide which call is most urgent.

Hold, Please

If you cannot take a call off hold after 90 seconds, check back and ask the caller whether he wants to continue holding. Again, wait for an answer before putting the call back on hold. If the hold lasts longer than three minutes, apologize to the caller for the delay. Offer to call the caller back as soon as you can.

Often, you'll be on the phone and have to answer another line. Ask the person you're talking with if she would mind holding. Wait for a reply before answering the second call. Explain to the second caller that you're on another line. Tell him that you need to finish that call. Don't handle the second call while the first caller waits *unless* the second call is:

- an emergency
- a long distance call that cannot be given to another worker
- a physician calling to speak with your physician

You'll often find yourself juggling phone calls and patients in the office. Use your judgment. If the call is going to be a long one, ask the caller to wait for a moment. Take care of the office patient first. Then return to the phone call.

INCOMING CALLS

Several types of routine calls will come into the office each day. Patients typically call the office to:

- make appointments
- report health emergencies
- seek medical advice
- request prescription refills
- obtain test results
- question a bill

Labs, health insurance providers, and other physicians also will commonly call the office throughout the day.

Many of the calls you receive will be from patients wanting to make appointments. Scheduling patient appointments is covered in Chapter 4.

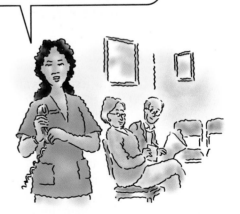

Be careful when talking on the phone in front of patients. Remember, all conversations with or about a patient are confidential.

Medical Emergencies

You must be able to tell the difference between panicked callers and true medical emergencies. First, try to calm the caller. Then ask specific questions about the patient's condition. The following conditions are true phone emergencies:

- chest pain
- severe pain of any kind
- difficulty breathing
- heavy bleeding
- loss of consciousness
- severe vomiting
- severe diarrhea
- fever above 102°

Put these calls through immediately. Some offices will assign a nurse to handle such calls.

Billing Inquiries

Your duties may include handling calls with questions about fees, bills, and insurance. Some callers may want to know what the physician charges for a certain service or treatment. Don't quote prices. Instead, tell the caller that charges depend on the type of examination needed and the tests that are performed.

Other calls will be from a patient's health insurance provider. The caller may want information about the patient. Be careful about giving out confidential patient information over the phone until you're sure of the caller's identity.

Test Results

Many test results are called into the physician's office before the written report is sent. Keep a supply of forms for recording such results on hand near the phone. Write the information down and put it on the front of the patient's chart for the physician to review. Later, the written report will be added to the chart when it's received.

If the test was ordered **stat,** this means the results are needed right away. Do not place phoned results of a *stat* test in the front of the chart. Instead, bring them to the physician's attention as soon as you get them. The physician must see the paperwork and sign or initial it first.

Patients often call the office for their test results. Many physicians allow their medical assistants to give favorable test results to patients. Your office will have a policy for handling these kinds of calls. Remember, however, that you may not give test results to anyone but the patient without the patient's permission. And never take it upon yourself to give a patient test results without the physician's permission.

If a patient's test results are seriously unsatisfactory, the physician will want to discuss them with the patient. If the results aren't too bad, the physician may ask you to speak with the patient instead.

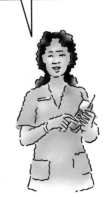

<u>Never</u> give bad test results to a patient unless the physician tells you to do so.

Progress Reports

Patients may be told to call the office in a few days to report how they're feeling. If the patient says she's better, take down her information, record it in her chart, and place the chart on the physician's desk for review.

Hospital, home health workers, and other health care providers also may call with progress reports on a patient. For example, a home care nurse may call to say that the patient's blood pressure is now within normal limits. A physical therapist may call to report that a patient's ability to use his arm is improving. Again, record the information in the chart and put it on the physician's desk for review.

The physician must speak with patients who do not report satisfactory progress. The patient's condition will determine how quickly the physician needs to talk with her. You should bring calls that report new symptoms or seriously worsening conditions to the physician's attention.

Prescription Refills

As a medical assistant, you can handle requests for refills of prescribed medicines if the chart shows that refills are permitted. If there's any doubt, tell the patient or pharmacist that you'll check with the physician and call back.

Other Routine Calls

Other kinds of calls you'll receive are:

- requests for referrals to other physicians
- questions from patients about the physician's instructions
- business calls related to running the office

Ask the physician which types of calls he wants to handle immediately, which he prefers to return later, and which should be transferred to other office staff.

Calls from other physicians are generally put through at once, unless your office's policy is to handle them differently. Physicians also get personal calls. Your supervisor will tell you what kinds of calls to put through and when you should take a message.

Unidentified Callers

Sometimes, a caller who asks to speak to the physician will not give you her name. Others may not wish to tell you the reason they are calling.

You should politely tell unidentified callers that the physician is busy and that you will be happy to take a message. If the caller persists, ask him to call again at a specific time the physician is available. Then alert the physician about the time of the expected call. Many unidentified callers may be salespeople.

Angry Callers

When a caller is angry, you must be careful to not lose your own temper. Try to calm the caller and assure her that you want to help. Listen carefully and take notes. If the caller is a patient and you cannot take care of the situation, tell her that you must talk to the physician or office manager. Offer to call her back. The physician may want to speak with the patient personally. Always tell the physician about complaints regarding fees or care.

TAKING PHONE MESSAGES

Taking phone messages will be a large part of your daily duties. You should have notepads designed especially for doing this. These can be either forms from an office supply company or forms designed especially for your office. Either way, they should be two-part forms with carbonless copies. This will give you a record of the messages you take each day and what you did on these calls.

At a minimum, the telephone message form should have places for you to write the following information:

- the caller's name
- the date and time of the call
- the phone number where the caller can be reached
- a short description of the caller's concern
- the person to whom you are giving the original part of the message form
- your initials so that the person who receives the message can check in with you if she has any questions

After you take a phone message, tell the caller when to expect a return call. Some physicians wait to return calls until the end of the day (except for emergencies, of course). Others return calls as they can throughout the day. Know your office's policy.

A note of all calls must be made in the patient's medical record. If you call the patient, write a summary of your conversation in the patient's chart. Some phone message forms are designed so that a copy of the message can be added to the chart in place of writing in it.

OUTGOING CALLS

You will be making, as well as answering, calls as a receptionist. You should prepare carefully for your calls. Have all the information you will need in front of you before you call the number. Plan ahead of time what you are going to say.

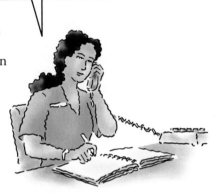

I'm sorry, sir, but I need to reschedule your appointment. Dr. Hobbs will be in surgery on Tuesday. Can you come at 9:00 Wednesday morning?

For example, suppose the physician has an emergency and you must call a patient to reschedule his appointment. Have the appointment book with you before you make the call. Be ready to explain why the physician is canceling. Also be prepared to offer a new appointment time.

Conference Calls

Your employer may ask you to set up a conference call. This is a call that puts three or more people on the line at the same time. Contact all the parties to the call in advance. This will ensure that they'll all be available at the planned time of the call. The exact procedure for making the call will depend on the kind of phone equipment your office has.

Outgoing Emergency Calls

When emergencies happen in the office, clinical staff may be busy trying to save a patient's life. They will direct you to call the local emergency medical service (EMS) to take the patient to a hospital.

Dial the EMS number. This number should be posted on every phone. Also, in most parts of the United States, you can reach EMS by dialing 911. Stay calm and speak clearly and slowly to the person who answers. Be prepared to provide:

- the patient's name, age, and gender. Age is especially important if the patient is an infant or a child. It allows the dispatcher to send the most appropriate responders.
- a brief description of the problem—for example, chest pain, the patient has stopped breathing, severe bleeding, etc.

- the level of service the physician is requesting—basic life support (BLS) or advanced life support (ALS). This also lets the dispatcher know how to respond.
- the street address of the office. Include any specific instructions for locating it. For example, "We're the Medical Office Group. Our office is on the fourth floor, third door on the left from the elevator."
- any added information, instructions, or requests the physician asks you to provide.

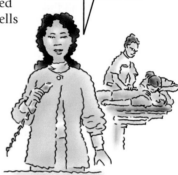

Never hang up when calling EMS until EMS tells you to do so.

After you give the information, if the dispatcher has additional questions, answer them. Ask the dispatcher when the ambulance is expected to arrive. Don't end the call until the dispatcher tells you to do so.

When you get off the phone, tell staff of EMS's estimated arrival time. Next, make sure the path through the office is clear for EMS to reach the patient. Then, reassure other patients in the reception area. If the patient has family members present, offer them reassurance and support. If an extra staff person is available, have him wait outside to flag down the EMS unit.

Written Communications

Good writing skills are important to medical assisting work. You'll be responsible for either writing or producing many types of documents. These might include:

- letters
- memos
- consultation reports
- agendas for meetings
- minutes from meetings
- instructions to patients

Poorly written letters and other documents will reflect badly on the office and on you. They also may affect a patient's quality of care.

WRITING A BUSINESS LETTER

You may be asked to write various kinds of letters. These may be sent to patients, insurance companies, drug companies, various other businesses, and other health care providers. Some examples include:

- letters welcoming new patients to the practice
- letters to patients about their test results
- consultation reports to other health care professionals
- explanations of treatments to insurance companies
- cover letters for transferring patients' records to other physicians
- explanations to patients about charges or other billing concerns
- thank-you letters to salespeople
- announcements of changes in office policies or services

Follow these three steps to create a professional business letter:

- prepare
- compose
- edit

Preparation

Good preparation is key when writing professional business letters. Preparation includes planning the letter's content and mechanics, as well as what the letter will look like.

Planning Content. Before you begin to write, plan your message. It may help to imagine yourself talking to the person who will receive the letter. Answering these questions also will help you prepare your message.

1. *Who is my reader?* Think about the reader's level of understanding. For example, letters to patients should be less technical and use fewer medical terms than letters to physicians.

2. *What do I want to say, and how shall I organize my message?* Briefly outline the information you want to include in the letter. Asking yourself *who, what, when, where, why,* and *how* may help you with this task.

3. *What do I want the reader to do?* If the reason for the letter is to ask for some action, you must tell the reader what to do. Be specific. If there's a deadline, state it. Enclosing an addressed and stamped reply envelope also may encourage the reader to act.

Planning Letter Mechanics. You should also plan what the letter will look like before you begin to type. This means deciding

Secrets for Success   ORGANIZING INFORMATION

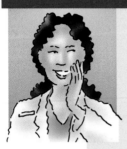

There are three basic ways to organize information—or the message—in written verbal communication:

- *Chronological.* Discuss items in sequence. Begin with the earliest date related to the information. Then go the next date, and the next, up to the most recent date. For example, this organization could be used in writing about the physician's background for the office's brochure for new patients.

- *Problem oriented.* Identify the problem, explain it, and provide instructions for correcting it. A letter to a patient reporting abnormal blood test results would first state the problem—a low potassium level, for example. Then it would explain the possible causes for this problem. Finally, it would suggest treatments and follow-up procedures.

- *Comparison.* Evaluate two or more items of information. For instance, if you were asked to evaluate two computer software packages the office was considering for purchase, you would use this approach.

Closer Look   FONT FACTS

The font chosen for a letter affects how it looks and how hard the words are to read. Here are some fonts that would be suitable for a business letter:

- This is 12-point Times New Roman.
- This is 10-point Times New Roman.
- This is 12-point Garamond.
- This is 12-point Arial.

Here are fonts and type sizes that would not be appropriate:

- This is 8-point Times New Roman.
- **This is 12-point Colossalis Black.**
- THIS IS 12-POINT COTTONWOOD.
- This is 12-point Tekton.
- **This is 12-point Impact.**

on the letter's margins, font, and template. The margin is the blank space between the type and the edge of the paper. A business letter might have margins of 1, 1.25, or 1.5 inches on the left and right sides of the page. Whatever margin you choose, it should be the same on each side.

The font is the type that will appear on the page. The font you choose will affect the way words look. The template is the letter's "skeleton." It determines how the letter is laid out on the page. Most computer word processing software has several templates to choose from. Pages 44–45 show a typical template and business letter.

Composition

When you compose your letter, state your message clearly and accurately. The message should be short and to the point. Avoid wordy phrases and long sentences.

A clear message ensures that your reader knows exactly what is expected. An unclear message leaves room for doubt.

Editing

After you've typed the letter, edit it. Review your writing for errors in the information and grammar. Editing is a key step in making your letter a success.

Check the following areas:

- accuracy of all information
- clarity in language used
- grammar
- spelling
- punctuation
- capitalization
- paragraphs appropriate in length
- logical organization and flow

Make any changes that result from this review.

If possible, print out a hard copy of the letter and have a coworker edit it. He may spot errors that you missed. He also can tell you if language that seemed clear to you may not be clear to someone else.

WRITING A MEMORANDUM

A memorandum, or memo, is used for written communication within the office. Often, memos are used for brief announcements. Memos are never sent to patients. They're less formal than letters.

Benjamin Matthews, M.D.
999 Oak Road, Suite 313
Middletown, Connecticut 06457
860-344-6000   ①

February 2, 2003 ②

Dr. Adam Meza
Medical Director   ③
Family Practice Associates
134 N. Tater Drive
West Hartford, Connecticut 06157

Re: Ms. Beatrice Suess ④

Dear Doctor Meza: ⑤

Thank you for asking me to evaluate Ms. Suess. I agree with your diagnosis of rheumatoid arthritis.
Her prodromal symptoms include vague articular pain and stiffness, weight loss and general malaise.
Ms. Suess states that the joint discomfort is most prominent in the mornings, gradually improving
throughout the day.

My physical examination shows a 40-year-old female patient in good health. Heart sounds normal,
no murmurs or gallops noted. Lung sounds clear. Enlarged lymph nodes were noted. Abdomen
soft, bowel sounds present, and the spleen was not enlarged. Extremities showed subcutaneous
nodules and flexion contractures on both hands.

⑥

Laboratory findings were indicative of rheumatoid arthritis. See attached laboratory data. I do
not feel x-rays are warranted at this time.

My recommendations are to continue Ms. Suess on salicylate therapy, rest and physical therapy.
I suggest that you have Ms. Suess attend physical therapy at the American Rehabilitation Center
on Main Street.

Thank you for this interesting consultation.

Yours truly,   ⑦

Benjamin Matthews, MD ⎞
                         ⎬ ⑧
Benjamin Matthews, MD   ⎠

BM/es ⑨

Enc. (2) ⑩

cc: Dr. Samuel Adams ⑪

The Parts of a Business Letter

A typical business letter has 11 parts. Each part is identified and described in the following numbered list. The numbers in the list correspond to the numbered part of the letter on the previous page.

1. *Letterhead.* The letterhead contains the name of the physician or practice, the address, and the telephone number. It also might contain the office fax number and e-mail address. It's often in color and it can be made part of the template itself.

2. *Date.* Place the date two to four spaces below the letterhead. Don't use abbreviations.

3. *Inside Address.* This is the name and address of the person who will be receiving the letter. Place the inside address four spaces below the date, unless a window envelope is being used. If that's the case, you may need to use different spacing to make the address visible through the window. If the letter is going to a business, insert the receiver's title as the second line, between the name and street address. The business name becomes the third line.

4. *Subject line.* The subject line is an optional line. If it's used, it appears on the third line below the inside address. It begins with *Re:* (the abbreviation for "regarding") followed by the subject.

5. *Salutation.* This is the greeting that starts the letter. Place the greeting two spaces below the inside address or the subject line. Make sure it contains the title and last name of the person receiving the letter—for example, *Dear Mr. Smith* or *Dear Ms. Jones.* If the letter is to a physician, write out *Doctor*—*Dear Doctor Smith*, not *Dear Dr. Smith.*

6. *Body.* This part of the letter contains the message. Single-space the body using a double space between paragraphs. Use letterhead only on the first page, if the body goes onto a second page.

7. *Closing.* The closing concludes the letter. Place the closing two spaces below the body. Capitalize only the first word. Insert a comma after the closing.

8. *Signature and name.* Type the name and title of the person signing the letter four spaces below the closing. If you're told to sign the letter, write the physician's name, followed by a slash mark and your name.

9. *Identification line.* The uppercase initials tell who composed the letter. The lowercase letters tell who prepared it. Like the subject line, this element is optional.

10. *Enclosure.* If something is included with the letter, use the initials *Enc.* to indicate that. If more than one document is included, show the total number in parentheses.

11. *Copy.* Use the letter *c* to show that a duplicate of the letter was sent somewhere else.

A sample memo is shown in reduced size on this page. In some ways, memos are like letters in style. But in many other ways, their style is different.

- *Heading.* Type the word *memorandum* across the top of the page.
- *To.* List the names of everyone who's going to receive the memo. If it's to an entire group, the group name can be typed instead of the individual names.
- *From.* Type the name and title of the person sending the memo.
- *Date.* Use the same rules as you do for letters when typing memo dates.
- *Subject.* Type a brief phase describing the purpose of the memo.
- The abbreviation *Re:* is sometimes used in place of *Subject.*
- *Body.* Insert the message of the memo.
- *Copy.* Use the same rules as you do for letters.

Memos don't use salutations and closings.

Writing a memo requires the same preparation, composition, and editing steps that letters do. Your computer software should have a memos template as well.

Franklin Dermatology Center
123 Main Street
Rockfall, Kansas
913-755-2600

Memorandum

To: All Medical Assistants
From: Patty Stricker, Office Manager
Date: 12/03/07
Re: Holiday time

Please notify me by December 10 of any requests you have for taking time off during Christmas or New Year's. Remember that holiday requests will be based on seniority. The office will be closed at noon on December 24. The office will be closed on the 25th and reopen on the 26th. The office will also close on December 31st at noon. The office will be closed on January 1, reopening on the 2nd.

If you have any questions, please e-mail me.

GUIDELINES FOR MEDICAL WRITING

Writing letters to medical professionals is similar to writing business letters. Some additional guidelines apply, however.

Accuracy

Medical writing requires even more accuracy and clarity than writing business letters does. Pay very careful attention to detail when you write medical letters and documents. Some of your letters will be placed in patients' permanent medical records. Mistakes here could cause injury or death, lawsuits, and harm to the physician's practice.

When the physician asks you to draft a letter about a patient, she may or may not give you notes to follow. Either way, your duty in typing the letter is to be as accurate as possible. You should question anything you're not sure about.

Here are some examples of inaccuracy in medical writing:

- The physician wrote, "The patient was started on the MVPP chemotherapy regime." You type MVP instead. These are two completely different treatments. MVPP is used for treating Hodgkin's lymphoma. MVP is used in treating lung cancer.

- The physician wrote, "Patient was told to take Dristan Cold tablets." You edited the physician's sentence and typed, "The patient had a cold and was told to take Dristan tablets." Dristan Cold contains a medication that plain Dristan does not.

- The physician wrote, "There is no reason for him to start radiation therapy at this time." But you typed, "There is reason for him to start radiation therapy at this time." This simple, one-word mistake could lead to a serious error in patient care.

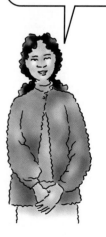

> Never edit a physician's writing unless you're absolutely sure the change will not affect the meaning.

Spelling

The spell-check feature in word processing programs can be a great help. But it has limitations. For instance, it will not find mistakes in which words are spelled correctly but are misused. Here's an example:

- "The patient's mucus was yellow."
- "The patient's mucous was yellow."

Mucus is a sticky secretion. Mucous is a membrane that secretes mucus. Both words are spelled correctly. The spell check will not flag either as an error. But the second sentence is wrong.

Also, be careful about plural forms of words. Making many medical terms plural can be tricky. For example, the plural of *bulla* (a blister) is not *bullas*. It is *bullae*.

Capitalization

Pay special attention to how words and abbreviations are capitalized. Never change how a word is capitalized unless you are told to do so. If you question a capitalization, mark a hard copy of the typed document with a question mark for the physician to answer.

For example, m-BACOD is a very different treatment from M-BACOD. Some other common medical terms with unusual capitalizations are: pH, RhoGam, rPA, ReoPro, and aVR.

Abbreviations and Symbols

Using abbreviations and symbols saves time in writing notes by hand. When typing medical information, however, spell out all abbreviations that are not part of everyday English. For example, PM is commonly understood as an indicator of time. But

Closer Look | COMMONLY MISSPELLED OR MISUSED MEDICAL TERMS

Here are some common medical words than can be misspelled and misused easily:

- anoxia and anorexia
- aphagia and aphasia
- bowl and bowel
- emphysema and empyema
- fundus and fungus
- lactose and lactase
- metatarsals and metacarpals
- mucus and mucous
- parental and parenteral
- postnatal and postnasal
- pubic and pubis
- rubella and rubeola
- serum and sebum
- uvula and vulva

NPO (meaning *nothing by mouth*) is not. Be familiar with the abbreviations and symbols that are used where you work. Most offices have a list of their approved ones.

Be careful when interpreting what abbreviations and symbols mean. Here are some examples of what can go wrong:

- The physician wrote "The patient had good BS." You assumed that BS meant bowel sounds. So you typed, "The patient had good bowel sounds." But what the physician meant by BS was *breath sounds*.

- Do not change < or > signs to *less than* or *greater than* unless you are sure what the symbol means. If the statement means, "Her hemoglobin is less than 13," and you mistakenly type, "Her hemoglobin is greater than 13," a treatment error could occur.

- The symbols for male ($\male$) and female ($\female$) are commonly used and understood. But you should replace them with words when writing a medical or business letter.

Numbers

Numbers one to ten should usually be spelled out in medical and business writing. There are exceptions, however.

- Units of measurement are always written as numbers, no matter how small—for example, 5 mg.

- Numbers referring to an obstetrical patient's condition are not spelled out. "The patient is gravida 3, para 2." Don't convert these numbers to words.

Be careful about placement of decimal points. There's a huge difference in dose between 1.25 mg and 12.5 mg of medication. Also, make sure you don't switch the order of numbers when you type them. Double-check for this very important kind of error. Suppose, for example, you typed, "The patient's red blood count was 5.1." But it was actually 1.5. A red blood count of 1.5 will not sustain life.

Sending Written Communications

Once a document has been typed, edited, and signed (if it's a letter), the next step is sending it. Most routine business letters are delivered by the United States Postal Service (USPS) through regular U.S. mail. Other means of sending documents are also available.

- *Overnight delivery by express mail.* The USPS offers this option. So do private delivery services such as FedEx and UPS.

- *Immediate delivery by electronic mail (e-mail) or fax.* These methods have drawbacks, however, despite their ease and speed. These limitations will be discussed below.

There are two key things to remember when sending any written communication:

- Make every attempt to ensure that confidential material is kept confidential. Mark the outside of such envelopes "confidential." This applies to all correspondence that contains information about a patient.
- Send letters only to known addresses. Include a return address on all mail, so that it can be returned if the person is no longer at that address.

USING U.S. MAIL

When written communications are sent by regular mail, USPS guidelines should be followed to prevent errors or delays in delivery.

Addressing Envelopes

Most letters will be sent in standard no. 10 business envelopes. Medical records, multipage test results, and some other reports and documents may be sent in larger, 9-by-12-inch mailing envelopes.

The USPS expects the delivery address to be in the center of the envelope. The equipment USPS uses to scan the envelope for address information does not recognize writing at its edges. Addresses on large envelopes can be printed on labels and then attached to the envelope. Addresses on business envelopes will usually be printed on the envelope itself.

On a no. 10 business envelope, type the address 12 spaces down from the top, centered on the face of the envelope. Single-space the address. Provide a line each for the addressee's name, name of the business (if any), street address, and the city and state. If you abbreviate the state name, use only the official USPS abbreviation.

The five-digit zip code must appear at the end of the line for city and state. You should include the four-digit expanded zip code whenever possible. Your computer software also may let you include a USPS PostNet bar code. This is generally inserted two or three lines below the address. This bar code will speed USPS handling of the envelope.

> Type addresses on labels or envelopes instead of writing them by hand. Typed envelopes give a professional image.

Place the return address in the upper left corner of the envelope. It should not exceed five lines, and it is also single-spaced. Many medical offices will have their return address preprinted on their envelopes.

Place special notations such as "personal" or "confidential" two lines below the return address. Put notations for hand canceling or special delivery in the upper right corner, below the postage. Don't put anything in the lower right corner of the envelope. The USPS uses that space for its bar codes.

ALL ABOUT ENVELOPES

Here are some other things to remember about envelopes:

- Be sure that any graphics on the envelope will not interfere with the ability of USPS electronic scanners to read the address.
- Don't use fancy fonts to type the address. This will interfere with the scanners' ability to read it.
- Don't use small type or dark envelopes. A white or tan envelope with black type is preferred.
- Don't use a # symbol in an address. If it cannot be avoided, the USPS recommends placing a space between the # symbol and the number.
- If you're using a window envelope, there should be an eighth-inch space between the edges of the window and the address showing from inside the envelope.

The Hands On procedures on page 60 give you step-by-step guidelines on how to properly fold a letter to go inside a standard business envelope and a window envelope.

Special Services

Sometimes, it's necessary for the office to have proof that a letter was sent. For example, the physician might decide to end her relationship with a patient. This requires that the patient be notified. You will read more about such legal procedures in Chapter 2. But they require that proof of notification be placed in the patient's medical record.

Proof of delivery is available from USPS by sending the letter by certified mail. This type of mailing requires an extra fee. But it provides a receipt that proves the letter was received. Place this receipt in the patient's record.

Private express-delivery companies such as FedEx and UPS offer tracking services that prove a letter was delivered. Using these companies is usually more expensive than certified mail, however. In addition, for an extra fee, you can require these companies to get someone at the address to sign for the letter before they will leave it. This provides proof the letter was received. But for legal purposes, proof it was delivered is enough in most cases.

FAXING DOCUMENTS

Facsimile machines (commonly called *fax* or *facs machines*) allow you to send and receive printed materials over a phone line. They're an easy and cheap way of sending records, physician's orders, test results, and other documents that must be received quickly.

When you send documents through a fax machine, include a cover sheet with them. The cover sheet is always the first page to be faxed. Most offices have a supply of printed cover sheets that you fill in for each fax. The cover sheet should contain the following information:

- name, address, telephone, and fax number of the office
- name of the person the fax is intended for
- telephone number of the receiver's fax machine
- date and time of the fax
- number of pages being sent (count the cover sheet too)
- confidentiality statement

Legal Brief THE CONFIDENTIALITY STATEMENT

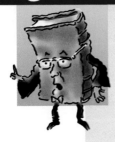

The confidentiality statement is necessary because the faxed information may be private. Patient test results, for example, are confidential and often are sent by fax. For legal purposes, a statement such as this one must appear on the cover sheet:

This sheet and any documents accompanying it are confidential. They are intended only for use by the person or entity named above. If you are not the intended recipient of these documents, you are hereby notified that any disclosure, copying, or distribution of this information is strictly prohibited. Notify the sender immediately by telephone.

Lack of confidentiality is one drawback of sending written communications by fax machine. You can't know for sure that it's the addressee who will actually pick up the fax at the other end.

Sometimes, when you fax documents to another fax machine, that machine may be busy sending or receiving other faxes. If this happens, your fax machine will keep redialing the number until it can send the fax. Don't use this feature, however, if unauthorized persons might have access to the documents while they are waiting to be faxed. Also, never leave documents in a fax machine unattended.

ELECTRONIC MAIL

Electronic mail, or e-mail, allows you to send files from your computer to another computer anywhere in the world. When communicating by e-mail, follow the same rules that you use when writing letters.

There are two ways of sending e-mails:

- You can send the document—a letter, for example—as an e-mail.

- You can send the document as an attachment to an e-mail.

Sending the document as an e-mail requires that you type it at the time you send it. If the document already exists in your computer somewhere, you can select it and attach it to a short e-mail letter that explains what is attached.

E-mail messages are often more secure than faxed materials. But confidentiality still cannot be guaranteed. Therefore, include a confidentiality statement in e-mails that contain confidential information. This is similar to the statement included on a fax cover sheet. You can easily adapt that sample cover sheet statement for use with e-mails.

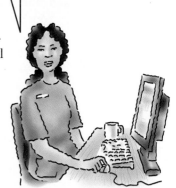

If you're attaching documents to an e-mail, open and look at them before you hit <u>send</u> to be sure you attached the correct documents.

Handling Incoming Mail

Part of your duties may be handling the incoming mail. Many types of mail will come into the office each day. They may include:

- advertisements
- bills from suppliers of goods and services
- consultation letters
- hospital communications and newsletters

- laboratory and radiology reports
- waiting room magazines
- professional journals
- literature from professional organizations
- samples of drugs and lab test kits
- payments from insurance companies and patients
- other patient correspondence

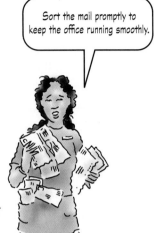

Sort the mail promptly to keep the office running smoothly.

OPENING AND SORTING MAIL

Some physicians may want you to sort, open, respond to, and file mail without their review. In other offices, all mail is handled only by the physician or office manager.

Most physicians will open and handle their own personal mail. Mail about patients, however, should be opened and dealt with as soon as possible.

Any mail marked "urgent" should be processed first, whether you're permitted to open it or not. Records, test results, and other patient-related materials are next in order. Ads, announcements, and other promotional materials are handled last.

Your office may have established policies and procedures for processing the daily mail. Some additional general procedures to follow that will help you do the job efficiently include the following:

1. Gather the needed equipment: a letter opener, paper clips, and a date stamp.

2. Open all letters and check for enclosures. Attach these with a paper clip to the letter. If the letter states there were enclosures and none were sent, contact the sender. Write on the letter that enclosures were missing and the name of the person you contacted.

3. Stamp all mail with the date it was received.

4. Sort the mail into categories and handle each according to office policy. In general, this will mean:
   - *Test results.* Attach test results to the patient's chart with paper clips and place the chart in a stack for the physician's review.
   - *Payments.* Record all checks and insurance payments and process them according to office policy.
   - *Advertisements.* Dispose of all advertisements unless you are told differently.

5. Distribute the mail to the proper staff member. Office policy will determine which member is responsible for each type of mail. The office manager may get all checks, for example. As a receptionist, you may be responsible for reception area magazines.

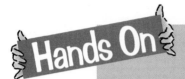

RECOGNIZING NONVERBAL CLUES

1-1

To be an active listener, you must be able to understand and deal with patients' nonverbal clues in addition to what they say. Here are some guidelines for getting the most out of nonverbal communications.

1. Maintain proper personal space, position, and posture. Your nonverbal communication is sending messages to the patient too.
   - Always look the patient in the face and be at eye level. Be aware of cultural differences when it comes to eye contact.
   - If the patient is sitting, you should sit too.
   - Use proper gestures.
   - Use touch, if the situation is appropriate

2. Observe the patient's facial expressions and posture. People's nonverbal messages can differ from their verbal ones.
   - If the patient's nonverbal clues differ from what he is saying, ask appropriate questions to clarify the mixed message.
   - If a patient's verbal response doesn't match with what you are seeing, tell the physician of your concerns.

Hands On   INTERVIEW SKILLS   1-2

Here are six things that will help you conduct effective interviews. These methods also can be used in other settings to improve communication.

1. *Reflect.* Repeat part of what you hear the person say and let him finish the sentence. For example, "You were saying that your back hurts you when you . . ." Reflecting encourages people to make further comments.

2. *Paraphrase.* Repeat what you've heard using your own words or phrases. Paraphrasing is a way of making sure you understood what was said. It usually begins by saying, "You're saying that . . ." or "It sounds as if . . ." followed by the rephrased content.

3. *Clarify.* Ask for examples when a patient gives you information that's confusing or hard to understand. For instance, ask, "Can you describe one of those dizzy spells?" The patient's example should help you better understand what he's saying.

4. *Ask open-ended questions.* Ask questions in ways that can't be answered *yes* or *no.* Begin questions with *what, when, how,* and *why.* When asking *why* questions—such as, "Why did you stop taking your medicine?"—be sure that your tone and manner aren't judgmental.

5. *Summarize.* Briefly review the information you have gathered. This gives the person a chance to correct wrong or unclear information. For example, suppose a patient reports stumbling often. You might summarize by saying, "You told me that you've been feeling dizzy and that you often stumble as you are walking."

6. *Allow silence.* Allow periods of silence. Silences can encourage people to talk more. Some people are uncomfortable with pauses in conversations. They feel the need to fill the silence with words. Silences also can be used to think about what's already been said.

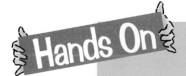

IDENTIFYING AND USING COMMUNITY RESOURCES   1-3

Patients sometimes will require help with problems beyond what your office or even the health care system is able to provide. Resources in the community may be available to meet these needs. Being aware of such resources is important to your role as a patient educator. Follow these guidelines to develop and use a list of community resources.

1. Determine what types of resources are most useful for the patients your office sees. This will largely depend on your office's medical specialty. But patients also may have needs that are not directly related to their medical problem. Services that might help with such needs are:
   - support groups and services for people with serious and potentially fatal diseases such as cancer or MS
   - support groups and services for people suffering from various types of abuse
   - services such as meals-on-wheels that help people who are ill or elderly
   - services for hearing- or sight-impaired people or those with mental disabilities

2. Create a list of sources from which to create a list of community services. Such a contact list might include:
   - social services departments at local hospitals
   - the local public health department
   - nursing home associations
   - local charities and church organizations
   - community service numbers in the local phone book
   - the Internet

3. Contact these resources to create a list of community services complete with addresses, email addresses, and phone numbers. Keep this list on your computer or, if it's too large, create a binder of information.

4. Provide patients with a printed list of specific services from your general list, according to their needs. Answer any questions they may have.

5. Offer to make the first contact for the patient. Recognize, however, that patients may prefer to do this themselves.

6. Document in the patient's chart that the information was provided.

Hands On   ORIENTING NEW PATIENTS   1-4

Educating new patients about the office and how it operates will help avoid confusion and future misunderstandings. Here are some steps to follow in orienting new patients to the office and its policies.

1. Gather needed materials such as the patient brochure or information about the practice and the physicians' business cards.

2. Give the patient these handouts. Point out the following information:
   * the physicians' names and specialties
   * the office's hours
   * the office's telephone numbers

3. Explain the office's policies and procedures on:
   * billing, payment, and filing insurance claims
   * making and canceling appointments
   * parking for patients

4. Ask if the patient has any questions.

5. Document in the patient's chart that the information was provided.

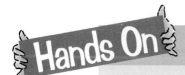 **HANDLING INCOMING CALLS**   1-5

Follow these steps to respond to incoming phone calls efficiently and professionally:

1. Have message pads and other needed supplies ready by the phone.

2. Answer the phone within two rings if possible.

3. Greet the caller with your name and the name of the office.

4. Identify the caller's reason for calling as soon as you can.

5. Triage the call. Prompt identification of emergency calls is important for good patient care.

6. Speak clearly and in a professional manner. Unhurried speech shows caring and will reassure the caller.

7. Clarify information with the caller. This will help prevent errors in communication.

8. Transfer the caller to the appropriate staff member if possible. If that person is not available, and if the call is not an emergency, offer to take a message.

9. Record any messages on a message pad. Include the caller's name, the date and time of the call, a number where the caller can be reached, a summary of the message, and the person to whom the form is routed. This practice creates a good record of phone communications with patients.

10. Give the caller an approximate time to expect a return call. This reassures the caller that the call will be handled properly.

11. Ask if the caller has any questions or needs other help. This confirms that the caller's needs have been met.

12. Allow the caller to hang up first. This assures that the caller has completed her communication.

13. Put the message in an appropriate place. This ensures the call has been handled correctly and that the intended staff member gets the information.

14. Complete the entire task within ten minutes. This provides prompt and efficient handling of incoming calls.

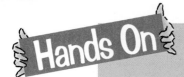

Hands On

FOLDING A LETTER FOR A BUSINESS ENVELOPE

1-6

Follow these steps to properly fold a letter for a no. 10 business envelope.

1. Place the letter face up on a flat surface. Using a flat surface helps you fold the letter neatly.

2. Fold the bottom third of the letter up and make a solid crease line. A solid crease creates a professional look.

3. Fold the top part of the letter down to within three-eighths of an inch of the first fold. Make a solid crease. This ensures that the second fold does not interfere with the first fold.

4. Place the letter in the envelope with the second fold at the top of the envelope. This allows the recipient to unfold the top part of the letter first.

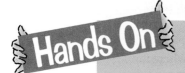

Hands On

FOLDING A LETTER FOR A WINDOW ENVELOPE

1-7

Follow these steps to properly fold a letter for a no. 10 window envelope.

1. Place the letter face up on a flat surface. Using a flat surface helps you fold the letter neatly.

2. Fold the bottom third of the letter up and make a solid crease line. A solid crease creates a professional look.

3. Fold the top part of the letter back and down to within three-eighths of an inch of the first fold. Make a solid crease. Folding the top down backwards allows the address on the letter to remain on the outside.

4. Place the letter in the envelope with the first fold at the top of the envelope. Turn the envelope over and make sure the recipient's address can be read through the envelope's window.

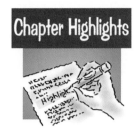

Chapter Highlights

- Communication is a process that involves the sending and receiving of verbal and nonverbal messages.
- Active listening and interviewing are important communication skills for working as a medical assistant.
- You will need to overcome many communication challenges to communicate with all patients. These include cultural and language differences as well as various patient impairments.
- Communicating with children and with angry, distressed, or grieving patients presents special challenges. You must use communication methods that are appropriate to the situation.
- A good attitude, professional appearance, and considerate manner send a positive message to patients about the care they receive.
- Working as a receptionist makes a medical assistant the most visible member of a medical office.
- The receptionist's main duties include preparing the day's patient charts, greeting arriving patients, managing the waiting room, and handling incoming phone calls.
- A good receptionist shows courtesy and diplomacy, even in difficult situations. She can triage phone calls effectively.
- Medical assistants need excellent written communication skills to write letters, memos, e-mails, and other documents.
- Careful attention to detail is very important, especially in medical writing. Errors in typing medical terms, numbers, and abbreviations can have serious consequences.
- A number of ways exist to send written communications after they are prepared.
- The opening, sorting, and handling of mail are among a medical assistant's duties in some medical offices.

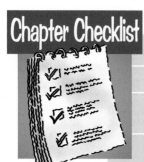

Chapter 2

LAW AND ETHICS FOR MEDICAL ASSISTANTS

Chapter Checklist

- Describe the two main branches of the American legal system
- Identify the three parts of a contract
- Explain the difference between implied contracts and expressed contracts
- List the items that must appear in a contract termination letter
- Explain informed consent, who may sign a consent form, and under what conditions informed consent cannot be given
- Describe the importance of the medical record as a legal document
- Identify and respond to issues of confidentiality
- Demonstrate knowledge of federal and state health care legislation and regulations
- Summarize the reasons for lawsuits against medical professionals and identify three possible defenses
- Explain the ways in which medical law applies to the medical assistant
- Identify the main ethical principles and issues in health care
- Perform within legal and ethical boundaries

The field of medicine and the field of law are closely linked. Their common bond is that both fields share a concern for people's well-being. During your career as a medical assistant, you'll be involved in many situations that have possible legal consequences. It will be important, both for you and your employer, that you act in lawful and ethical ways. You'll learn about ethics in this chapter. You'll also learn how the law applies to the practice of medicine and to everyday activities in your medical office.

The Law

Literally thousands of laws govern our daily lives and actions. We're familiar with many of these laws, such as traffic laws. However, most people have never heard of many other laws. But the following truth remains: "Ignorance of the law is no excuse."

Many of these important laws apply to the health care workplace. As a medical assistant, you must have a basic understanding of these laws. Knowledge of the laws will help you follow legal guidelines.

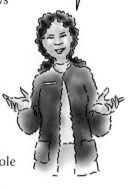

Knowing the law helps you protect your patients, your employer, and yourself.

PLAY BY THE RULES

Laws are rules of conduct that government creates. They exist to ensure the rights of all Americans. We depend on laws and the legal system that enforces them to protect us from the wrongdoings of others.

As a medical assistant, you need to understand the legal aspects of relationships with patients. You must be clear about your legal duties. You must also know your role and responsibilities in acting on behalf of the physician.

In the practice of medicine, charges of wrongdoing can arise in even the best of patient relationships. Many kinds of wrongdoing can take place in the typical medical office. Just one simple mistake can harm a patient and result in a lawsuit.

I'LL SEE YOU IN COURT

Two kinds of law exist in the United States—public law and private law, or **civil law.**

Public Law

Public law deals with issues between the government and citizens. There are four basic types of public law:

- *Constitutional law* is often called the law of the land. The U.S. government has a constitution that defines and limits

its powers. Each state also has its own constitution. U.S. laws must not contradict the U.S. Constitution. A state's laws cannot contradict either its state constitution or the U.S. Constitution.

- *Criminal law* deals with public safety. Laws against murder, theft, and sexual assault are examples of criminal laws. Medical assistants generally don't need to worry about breaking criminal laws in the workplace. However, practicing medicine without a license is a violation of criminal law. That's one reason never to treat patients without a physician's orders!

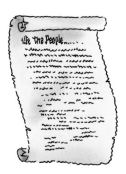

Two examples of constitutional law are laws on abortion and on civil rights.

- *Administrative law* is made up of the rules issued by government agencies. For example, the U.S. Food and Drug Administration (FDA) and a state's board of medical examiners both make rules affecting health care professionals.

- *International law* concerns treaties between nations. Trade agreements among countries are also part of international law.

Civil Law

Civil law is also called private law because it focuses on issues between private citizens. The medical profession is mainly involved with three types of civil law: contract law, commercial law, and tort law.

- *Contract law* and *commercial law* concern the rights and duties of people who enter into contracts. The physician-patient relationship falls under contract law.

- *Tort law* deals with righting the wrongs someone suffers because another person failed to carry out a legal duty. Tort law is the basis of most lawsuits against health care workers.

Tort law is the type of law that most often affects medical assistants as well as other health care professionals.

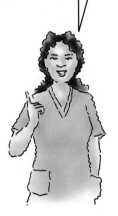

MEDICAL LEGAL CASES

Malpractice is an action by a health care professional that harms a patient. In the past 50 years, there's been a huge increase in the number of medical malpractice cases brought to court. A government investigation found four main reasons for the rise in claims of malpractice.

- *Scientific advances.* As new medical technology is available, the risk of complications from these procedures rises. This increases the chances of a lawsuit.

Closer Look | MALPRACTICE AWARDS

The amount of money awarded in lawsuits for malpractice has increased. Here are just two of the ways this trend has affected health care.

- Malpractice insurance is more expensive for health care professionals.
- Patients pay more for insurance policies that offer less coverage.

- *Unrealistic expectations.* Some patients expect miracle cures and file lawsuits when their recovery isn't as expected, even if the physician isn't at fault.
- *Economic factors.* Some patients view lawsuits as a way to get quick cash.
- *Poor communication.* Studies show that patients are more likely to sue when they don't feel a bond with their physician.

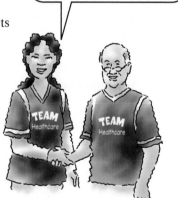

Nearly all dissatisfied patients will give you another chance if you move quickly to resolve their complaints.

The Physician-Patient Relationship

The relationship between a patient and his or her physician is a legal contract.

CONTRACTS

A **contract** is a special type of agreement between two or more parties. Agreements become contracts when three conditions are present:

- Offer: Someone offers to do something.
- Acceptance: Both parties agree to the terms.
- Consideration: Something of value is exchanged.

Three . . . Two . . . One . . . Contract

A contract that is made orally or in writing is called an **expressed contract.** In the American legal system, however, contracts can occur without any oral or written agreement. This type of contract is called an **implied contract.**

- *Offer* occurs when a patient calls the office to request an appointment.
- *Acceptance* takes place when you make the appointment for the patient.
- *Consideration* is present because in return for a fee, the physician will treat the patient.

Congratulations! You have just made a contract!

The patient arrives for the appointment and is seen by the physician. It's *implied* that because the patient came in on his own and requested care, he wants this physician to care for him. By taking care of the patient, the physician *implies* that she accepts this responsibility. By accepting the physician's services, the patient *implies* that he'll pay, even if the fee was never discussed.

RIGHTS AND RESPONSIBILITIES

Each party to a contract has certain rights, as well as certain duties or responsibilities. The rights and responsibilities of the parties in a physician-patient relationship are outlined in the accompanying table.

Termination

In most cases, the contract ends when the patient's treatment is complete and the physician has been paid. The patient also may end the contract at any time. However, if the patient still seeks treatment and the physician wishes to end the contract, the physician must follow specific legal procedures to end the physician-patient relationship.

The physician may terminate the contract with the patient in the following circumstances:

- The patient does not keep appointments.
- The patient refuses to follow orders.
- The physician has personal reasons for wishing to end the physician-patient relationship.

To end the contract, the physician must send the patient a letter that includes:

- a statement that the physician intends to end the relationship
- an explanation of the reasons for this action
- a termination date that is at least 30 days from the date the letter is received
- a statement that the patient's medical records will be transferred to another physician at the patient's request

The Physician-Patient Relationship

Rights in the Physician-Patient Relationship	Responsibilities in the Physician-Patient Relationship
The Patient's Rights: • To choose a physician • To decide whether to begin treatment • To set limits on treatment • To know in advance what the treatment will be • To know in advance the treatment's expected effects and possible dangers	The Patient's Responsibilities: • To give accurate information about his or her symptoms • To provide a complete and accurate medical history • To follow the physician's instructions • To pay the physician for services provided
The Physician's Rights: • To limit the practice to a certain specialty or location • To refuse to serve new patients • To refuse to serve current patients with new problems • To change policies after giving fair notice of the change	The Physician's Responsibilities: • To respect the patient's confidential information • To inform the patient about his or her condition, treatment, and chances for recovery • To give complete and accurate information • To provide reasonable skill, experience, and knowledge in treating the patient • To treat the patient as long as the condition requires, or until the contract is withdrawn • To obtain informed consent before performing procedures • To caution against unneeded or undesirable treatment

- a strong recommendation that the patient seek any additional medical care that may be required

The termination letter must be sent by certified mail with a return receipt requested. Place the return receipt and a copy of the letter in the patient's record.

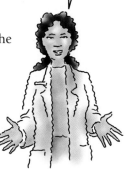

Send all termination letters by certified mail with a return receipt requested.

Abandonment

If the physician doesn't terminate the contract properly, the patient can sue him for **abandonment.** Abandonment occurs when the physician ends the relationship without proper notice while the patient still needs treatment.

The following situations also are abandonment:

- The physician doesn't see the patient as often as the condition requires.

- The physician incorrectly tells the patient that no more treatment is needed.

- The physician does not arrange for another doctor to care for the patient when the physician must be away.

CONSENT

Consent is agreement to something. The law requires that patients consent to being treated, examined, or even touched by the physician and anyone assisting him or her. No treatment can take place without some form of consent. Consent may be obtained in two ways:

- *verbally* in a spoken or written statement
- *nonverbally* by the patient's actions or behavior

Implied Consent

In many cases, a patient's actions indicate his or her consent to treatment. For example, a patient who pulls up his sleeve to receive an injection is informally and nonverbally agreeing to the injection. This type of consent is called **implied consent** because the patient's actions *imply* that he agrees to be treated.

Another kind of implied consent occurs in many emergencies. If a patient's problem is life threatening and she isn't able to give verbal permission for treatment, it's assumed that she would agree if she could.

In ordinary circumstances, implied consent is only used if treatment is unlikely to put the patient at risk.

Expressed and Informed Consent

The physician must obtain the patient's written, informed consent whenever the treatment involves the following:

- an invasive procedure, such as surgery
- the use of experimental drugs
- possibly dangerous procedures such as stress tests
- any significant risk to the patient

Informed consent means that the patient is aware of the benefits and risks of the treatment and its alternatives, and he voluntarily agrees to be treated. Generally, a patient gives informed consent by signing a form stating that he's aware of all these things. In getting informed consent, the physician must communicate with the patient in a way that the patient can understand.

As a medical assistant, you'll often be signing consent forms as a witness to the patient's signature. The consent form a patient signs must be in a language he or she speaks.

SIGNING CONSENT FORMS

A patient should *not* be asked to sign a consent form in these situations:

- The patient doesn't understand the treatment.
- The patient has unanswered questions about the treatment.
- The patient is unable to read the consent form.

Never try to force or convince a patient to sign a consent form if he or she doesn't want to. A patient should not feel pressured to sign the form.

Who May Sign a Consent Form? An adult (in most states anyone age 18 or older) may sign a consent form if he or she is mentally competent and not under the influence of any medication or other substances. Legal guardians also may sign consent forms. A **legal guardian** is someone appointed by a judge to act for a person who's not legally able to make decisions.

Most often, patients will have legal guardians because in some way they are not mentally competent. Sometimes patients who are **minors**—in most states someone under age 18—will have a legal guardian, too.

A minor may sign a consent form only if he or she is:

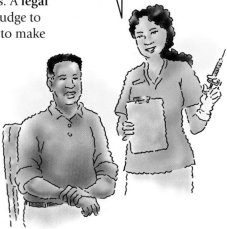

In many states you must get a patient's informed consent before performing an HIV test.

- in the armed forces
- seeking treatment for a contagious disease (including sexually transmitted diseases)
- requesting information about birth control or abortion
- requesting information about counseling for drug or alcohol abuse
- pregnant
- an emancipated minor

Secrets for Success COMPARE AND CONTRAST

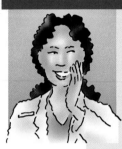

Here's a tip to boost your study skills: learn to compare and contrast.

- You'll notice that many topics in your study of medical assisting are related to other topics.
  - To *compare* topics, look for ways they're alike.
  - To *contrast* them, notice how they're different.

This strategy helps you see relationships between topics and understand both better.

- Let's apply this tip to the topic of consent.
  - If you compare informed consent and implied consent, you'll find that in both, the patient agrees to be treated.
  - In contrasting them, you'll find that in one case the consent is given in writing and in the other it's not.

Consider this: On page 65, you read about patients suing when their treatment didn't turn out as expected. Patient consent is sometimes an issue in such lawsuits. Do you think having the patient's informed consent or implied consent would be better for the physician in such a case? Comparing and contrasting informed and implied consent helps you to see the correct answer to this question.

In most other cases, the minor's parent or legal guardian must sign the consent form to treat a minor.

Health Care Surrogates. Health care surrogates also may sign consent forms in certain circumstances. A **health care surrogate** is a person the patient has chosen to make health care decisions for him if he or she is unable to make them. The patient has signed a document called a **durable power of attorney for health care** to name this person as health care surrogate.

An emancipated minor is someone who's under the age of majority (age 18 in most states) but who's married or self-supporting and is responsible for his or her debts.

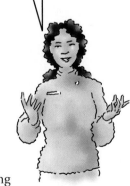

I Refuse to Consent!

A patient has the right to refuse treatment for any reason. If a patient refuses a treatment, the physician has the legal right to refuse to continue treating the patient. For example, a physician can refuse to perform surgery on a patient who won't receive blood if it's needed.

Some patients may refuse certain treatments because of their religious beliefs. Others may base their decision on personal preferences. For instance, a patient might refuse a treatment because of a negative effect it could have on her lifestyle. Patients who refuse treatment must be asked to sign a form stating that they have been advised of the treatment's benefits and risks, as well as the risks of not having it.

If parents refuse to allow the treatment of a minor, the courts may get involved. A judge may then give the consent needed for the child's treatment. The physician and her staff should follow any legal advice very carefully in such situations. The physician should also keep very detailed records of the case.

MEDICAL RECORDS

A patient's medical record is a legal document. Although the record itself belongs to the physician, the information in it belongs to the patient. Patients have a right to their medical information. They also have a right to deny the sharing of this information. There are several major exceptions to this second right, however.

Requests for medical records are common. Aside from the patient, other people who may need information from a medical chart are:

Whenever someone refuses treatment, thorough records must be kept to help protect the office from possible legal problems in the future.

- other health care providers
- a patient's insurance company
- certain government agencies

In general, you can legally provide a patient's medical information to these requesters without the patient's permission.

LEGALLY REQUIRED DISCLOSURES

Health care providers have a legal duty to report certain events to government authorities, even without the patient's consent. These circumstances are known as **legally required disclosures.** Health care providers must report to the department of public health in the situations discussed on this page and page 74.

Vital Statistics Reports

All states keep records of births, deaths, marriages, and divorces. The vital statistics records that concern health care providers are:

- *Birth certificates.* Most states require physicians to report live births they have attended. They must fill out, sign, and file a birth certificate.
- *Death certificates.* These must be signed by a physician. The time and cause of death must be included on them.
- *Stillbirth reports.* Some states have separate forms for reporting babies that were not alive when they were delivered. Other states use regular death certificates.

Medical Examiner's Reports

All states also have laws requiring that certain kinds of deaths be reported to the local medical examiner's office. These situations usually include:

- a death from an unknown cause
- a death from a suspected criminal or violent act
- a death within 24 hours of admission to a hospital
- a death in which a physician was not present at the time of, or during a reasonable period before, the death

Infectious or Communicable Diseases

An **infectious disease** is a disease that is caused by some organism that gets into the body, such as a virus, bacteria, or a parasite. A **communicable disease** is a disease that can spread from one person to another.

State law usually requires that certain infectious or communicable diseases be reported to the local health department. Exact requirements vary from state to state. In general, however, there are three general types of reports.

- *Telephone reports.* These are required for diphtheria, cholera, meningococcal meningitis, and plague. Reports of these diseases usually must be made within 24 hours after they are diagnosed. Telephone reports must always be followed by written reports.
- *Written reports.* These are required for hepatitis, leprosy, malaria, rubeola, polio, rheumatic fever, tetanus, and tuberculosis. Sexually transmitted diseases (STDs) must also be reported. Reports are usually required within 3 days of diagnosis.
- *Trend reports.* These are made when your office notes a high number of any infectious disease cases.

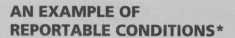

Closer Look

AN EXAMPLE OF REPORTABLE CONDITIONS*

Different states have different laws about reportable conditions. The following list from North Carolina contains only some of the diseases and conditions that have been declared to be dangerous to the public health and are hereby made reportable within the specified time period once the disease or condition is reasonably expected to exist.

acquired immunity deficiency syndrome (AIDS)—7 days

anthrax—24 hours

chlamydial infection (laboratory confirmed)—7 days

cholera—24 hours

diphtheria—24 hours

E. coli infection—24 hours

encephalitis—7 days

food-borne disease, including but not limited to
  Clostridium perfringens, staphylococcal, and *Bacillus cereus*—24 hours

gonorrhea—24 hours

hepatitis A or B—24 hours

hepatitis non-A, non-B—7 days

human immunodeficiency virus infection (HIV)
  confirmed—7 days

Lyme disease—7 days

malaria—7 days

measles (rubeola)—24 hours

meningitis, pneumococcal or viral—7 days

mumps—7 days

*Excerpt from the *North Carolina Administrative Code*

Vaccine Information Statements

Federal law requires health care providers who give certain vaccines and other injections to notify the U.S. Department of Health and Human Services (DHHS) in some situations. They must report when any side effects occur that are listed on the vaccine information sheet that the manufacturer includes in the package.

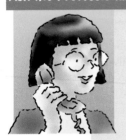

Ask the Professional — LEGALLY REQUIRED DISCLOSURES

Q: *I took a call from an angry patient today. He demanded to know why we told the health department we were treating him for an STD. The health department called him yesterday, wanting the name and phone number of his girlfriend. He was really mad! He said we had no right to turn him in like that. He was yelling so loud that my ear hurt. It was so unpleasant. How can I handle situations like this better in the future?*

A: To help prevent angry calls such as this one, always advise patients who have reportable conditions of this requirement. Tell them why such reporting is necessary, who will receive the information, and what forms will be used. Assure them that every effort will be made to protect their privacy. But also tell patients if they should expect any follow-up. For example, the health department will contact a patient with a reported STD to get the names of his or her sexual partners so they can be notified. Patients who are educated about legally required disclosures will usually be more accepting of your need to make these reports.

The health care provider must also put the following information in the patient's medical record:

- the date the vaccine was given
- the manufacturer of the vaccine
- the manufacturing lot number of the vaccine
- any unfavorable reactions to the vaccine
- the name, title, and address of the person who gave the vaccination

Abuse and Neglect

Each state has its own requirements about abuse, neglect, and other mistreatment. Generally, the mistreatment of someone who isn't able to protect himself or herself must be reported. The requirement applies to children in all states. Many states also include people who are elderly or mentally incompetent in this category.

Child Abuse. Abuse is believed to be the second most common cause of death in children under age 5. Federal law requires that threats to a child's physical and mental well-being be reported. The law shields health care workers, teachers, and social workers who report suspected child abuse. They are not identified to parents, and they are protected from being sued for reporting their suspicions.

If you suspect a child is being abused, you should tell the physician about your suspicions. The physician will file the actual report. The authorities will follow up by investigating the situation.

If you suspect child abuse, first tell the physician your suspicions. For assistance in reporting suspected child abuse, call the 24-hour national hotline at 800-4 A CHILD (800-422-4453).

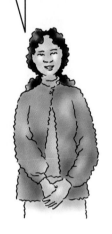

Spousal Abuse. Domestic violence is a widespread problem in the United States. Women and children especially are the victims of abuse. Women who depend on their abuser financially often feel trapped and see no way out of their situation. It will help you to keep the following tips in mind:

- Record any information gathered in the patient interview that may suggest abuse.
- Record any other signs of abuse you may observe.
- Tell the physician about your observations and suspicions.

Many communities have safe places for victims of domestic abuse. It is helpful to be aware of these services in your community.

Elder Abuse. The United States is also experiencing a rise in the abuse of elderly people. Elder abuse can involve both mistreatment and neglect—that is, not providing needed care. Observe elderly patients and pay close attention to the information they provide. If you suspect mistreatment or neglect, alert the physician. Also be aware of support groups that may exist in your community for people who provide care to the elderly.

For more information about domestic violence, call the National Domestic Violence Hotline at 1-800-799-SAFE.

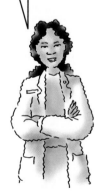

Violent Injuries

Health care providers also have a legal duty to report suspected violations of criminal law. Injuries to patients that were caused by weapons must be reported to authorities. Suspected assaults, rapes, and attempted suicides also must be reported.

Closer Look  OTHER REPORTS

There are other conditions that must be reported. They include:

- *Cancer.* This disease must be reported when it is diagnosed. This helps health officials track certain types of cancers and identify possible causes in the environment.
- *Epilepsy.* Some states require that epilepsy, a condition that causes seizures, be reported to motor vehicle departments.
- *Hyperthyroidism.* When discovered in infants, this is also a reportable condition in some states.
- *Phenylketonuria (PKU).* All states require that newborns be tested for phenylketonuria (PKU), which can cause mental retardation. Some states require positive PKU tests to be reported to the health department. This helps make sure that proper follow-up and care is provided to prevent serious problems for the infant.

Laws That Apply to Health Care Professionals

A variety of federal and state laws apply to the work that goes on in a heath care setting.

LAWS THAT REGULATE HEALTH CARE WORK

Medical professionals can be licensed, registered, or certified. Laws such as medical practice acts and nursing practice acts control licensing. Each state has its own laws in these areas. The laws usually state what kinds of activities are included in the practice of the profession. They also set the standards and procedures for being licensed to practice the profession.

Licensing

A licensed medical professional must have a license in each state where he or she

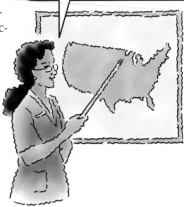

Every state has laws covering patient care, insurance billing, and other subjects related to the practice of medicine. Each state's laws also cover licensing.

works. Each state issues its own licenses and sets the qualifications to obtain and renew them. Most license holders are limited to specific duties. They also must practice their profession according to certain guidelines.

In most states, a licensed professional may lose his or her license, either temporarily or permanently, for any of the following reasons:

- *Criminal offenses.* This includes conviction for robbery, rape, and most other serious crimes.
- *Fraud.* This may include filing false insurance claims, falsifying medical records, and **fee splitting**—sharing fees for referring a patient to another professional.
- *Unprofessional conduct.* Examples include invasion of a patient's privacy, excessive use of alcohol, or use of illegal drugs.
- *Incompetence.* This is often a hard charge to prove. The most common examples are insanity, senility, or other mental defects.

As a medical assistant, it's your ethical duty to report illegal, unprofessional, or incompetent behavior. There's more about ethics and your duties as a medical assistant later in this chapter.

Registration and Certification

The term *registered* generally means that a professional has met basic requirements and has been approved to perform certain tasks in a state. The requirements and the approval come from a government body.

A professional organization, rather than the government, controls **certification**. The organization that issues the certifi-

---

Closer Look   FRAUD

Fraud is one of the most common reasons for losing a license. Examples include:

- advertising a cure that doesn't work
- guaranteeing the success of a treatment
- falsifying your credentials
- falsifying information on a bill to a patient's health insurance plan

cate sets the requirements for certification. Certification is a voluntary process. It generally isn't required to work in the health care professions. However, many physicians and clinics prefer to hire certified employees. Certification assures employers that applicants have met basic standards for the jobs they will perform.

The Certified Medical Assistant (CMA) and Registered Medical Assistant (RMA) are nationally recognized certifications. (Despite its title, the RMA is a certification.) They do not require any action when moving from one state to another. Most states do not require certification to work as a medical assistant. However, a few require you to pass a test or complete a short course before performing certain clinical duties.

GOOD SAMARITAN LAWS

Each state has a Good Samaritan Act. These laws are designed to encourage people to give emergency medical care without fear of being sued if something goes wrong. The laws vary from state to state. Some states set higher standards on the aid of trained professionals than for care provided by other citizens.

Closer Look   DETERMINING YOUR DUTIES

Because medical assistants are not licensed or registered, your potential range of activities is fairly broad. Keep these things in mind:

- Within certain limits, your employer has the power to set the duties you'll perform.

- These limits generally depend on the laws in your state that define the practice of medicine, nursing, and other health care professions. For example, some states allow only an MD, RN, or other licensed professional to give medications.

- Of course, you also must obey all laws regarding medical assisting or medical practice that may exist in the state where you work.

In general, good Samaritan laws protect you from lawsuits if the following conditions are met:

- The victim, if conscious, seeks or is willing to accept aid.
- You behave in a way that any reasonable person would in the situation.
- You do not act recklessly or intentionally perform any bad acts.
- You do not expect or receive payment for your help.

It's important to understand that good Samaritan laws do *not* cover your work as a medical assistant. They'll protect you only if you give someone aid when you're not on the job. Liability and malpractice insurance policies are available to protect you from lawsuits in work situations.

Of course, your best protection is to understand your ethical obligations and scope of duties as a medical assistant. You can find more information about your legal protection as it relates to your duties later in this chapter.

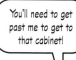

Remember, you should provide care as the law allows. Talk with the physician if you have questions.

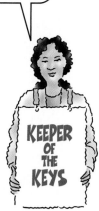

CONTROLLED SUBSTANCES ACT

The Drug Enforcement Administration (DEA) enforces the Controlled Substances Act of 1970. This federal law regulates the manufacture, distribution, and dispensing of narcotics and other drugs with a high potential for abuse. It's designed to decrease the illegal use or overuse of these substances. The law requires that physicians who use controlled substances to treat patients be registered with the DEA.

Here are some other requirements:

- All controlled substances must be kept in a locked cabinet that is out of patients' view.
- The keys to the cabinet must be kept secure.
- Controlled substances must be ordered on a special order form provided by the DEA.
- Orders and use of controlled substances must be recorded. These records must be kept for at least two years and must be available for inspection by the DEA at any time.
- The special prescription pads used for prescribing controlled substances must remain in a safe place at all times.

You should immediately report the theft of controlled substances or prescription pads to the DEA as well as to the local police. A list of controlled substances is shown in the accompanying table.

Schedule of Controlled Substances

The DEA groups controlled drugs into five classes or "schedules," according to their potential for abuse.

Schedule of Controlled Substances		
Schedule	**Description**	**Examples**
Schedule I	• High potential for abuse • Has no commonly accepted medical use in U.S. • No safety standards for medical use	• Heroin • Marijuana • Lysergic acid diethylamide (LSD)
Schedule II	• High potential for abuse • Abuse can lead to severe psychological or physical dependence • Have accepted medical use, but with strict limits • Require a written prescription and cannot be refilled • Prescription can be called in to pharmacist by physician only in emergencies, followed by written prescription within 72 hours • Cannot be called in by other health care workers	• Amphetamine • Cocaine • Codeine • Hydrocodone • Morphine • Oxycodone • Opium • Phencyclidine (PCP) • Ritalin • Seconal
Schedule III	• Have limited potential for psychological or physical dependence • Can be called in to pharmacist by physician • Can be refilled up to five times in a six-month period	• Anabolic steroids • Paregoric • Tylenol with codeine
Schedule IV	• Have lower potential for abuse than Schedule II or III drugs • Can be called in to pharmacist by medical office employee • Can be refilled up to five times in a six-month period	• Darvon • Librium • Phenobarbital • Valium • Xanax
Schedule V	• Have lower potential for abuse than Schedule IV drugs	• Lomotil • Cough medicines containing codeine

EMPLOYMENT AND SAFETY LAWS

A number of federal laws protect the health and welfare of employees in the workplace.

Civil Rights Act of 1964

Title VII of the Civil Rights Act of 1964 protects employees from discrimination in the workplace. Employers cannot hire, fire, or set pay for employees on the basis of gender, religion, race, or national origin. Nor can an employer provide working conditions or privileges based on these factors. The Equal Employment Opportunity Commission (EEOC) enforces this law and looks into possible violations.

Over the years, Title VII has been expanded to ban discrimination based on age and family status. For example, an employer can't ask a job applicant if he or she is married or has children.

Employers may legally ask about criminal convictions, however. They also can require a criminal records check and a drug screen of applicants because these precautions help ensure the safety of patients.

Sexual Harassment. Another way that Title VII has been expanded is to outlaw sexual harassment. The EEOC defines sexual harassment as unwelcome sexual advances in the workplace. It also includes sexual remarks or physical conduct that create an environment other workers find offensive. Every medical office should have in place standards of proper conduct and policies for handling complaints of sexual harassment.

Americans with Disabilities Act

The Americans with Disabilities Act (ADA) outlaws discrimination against people with disabilities. In the workplace, that includes hiring, firing, promotion, and compensation practices. The law also applies to training, benefits, and all other privileges of employment.

> Make sure you know what kind of behavior constitutes sexual harassment. If problems arise, follow your office's policies to resolve the matter.

There are laws to protect people with disabilities that limit their major life activities. People with AIDS or HIV-positive status, a history of mental illness, or a history of cancer are also covered.

The ADA allows employers to set physical standards for certain jobs, however. For example, a medical assistant might need a certain level of vision to see the dials on equipment.

All employers with 15 employees or more must comply with the ADA. The law requires them to provide such things as:

- special parking places close to the door
- ramps and elevators when curbs and steps are present
- bathrooms and break areas designed for people with disabilities
- work counters low enough for someone in a wheelchair

Occupational Safety and Health Act

The Occupational Safety and Health Act requires employers to provide a safe workplace for employees. The law created the Occupational Safety and Health Administration (OSHA) to set standards for workplace safety.

Special OSHA rules apply to medical environments. Some of the most important ones protect workers from **pathogens** in the blood and body fluids of patients. Pathogens are organisms that can cause disease. OSHA defines body fluids as:

- saliva
- semen
- vaginal secretions
- synovial fluid (from joint spaces)
- pleural fluid (from the lungs)
- pericardial fluid (from the heart)
- cerebrospinal fluid (from the spinal cord)
- amniotic fluid (from the uterus of a pregnant woman)
- any body fluid, such as emesis (vomit) or urine, that is visibly contaminated with blood

OSHA regulations require health care workers who have direct contact with patients to use protective equipment that includes:

- gloves
- gowns
- face masks

The Clinical Laboratory Improvement Amendments of 1988 (CLIA) provide rules related to laboratory safety. OSHA employees may conduct inspections of workplaces. Violations of its rules can result in fines or other penalties.

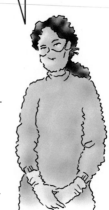

Personal protective equipment includes gloves, a gown, and a face mask. Your training will include further study of safety matters and how to protect yourself in the workplace.

HIPAA

You first read about the Health Insurance Portability and Accountability Act of 1996 (HIPAA) in Chapter 1. You will come across it again in nearly every chapter of this book. This is because HIPAA has brought major change to the health care industry.

Congress passed HIPAA, in part, to improve the efficiency of the nation's health care system. One way to do this was to require that insurance claims be submitted electronically, by computer. You will read

Legal Brief HIPAA

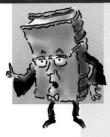

Here are just some of the ways HIPAA has affected the job of a medical assistant.

- It requires that the billing of patients' health insurance for the costs of treatment be done by computer.
- It set requirements for how treatments and procedures are identified on bills submitted to health insurance.
- It changed how private information in patients' medical records is handled and protected.
- It established guidelines for the security of patient information on the computer and in other places.

more about submitting health insurance claims in Chapter 8. HIPAA also changed how these claims are coded. You will learn about coding medical treatments and procedures in Chapter 7.

Congress realized that some of these changes could threaten the privacy of patients' health information. So HIPAA required the U.S. Department of Health and Human Services (DHHS) to make rules for patient privacy and computer security that health care facilities must follow.

You'll read about the requirements for computer security in Chapter 3. You already read in Chapter 1 about the privacy notice HIPAA requires you to give patients on their first office visit.

Medical Law

Imagine that a medical assistant is giving a patient a heat treatment for aching muscles. Suppose that she burns the patient's arm because the equipment did not work properly. A **tort** has occurred. A tort is a wrongful act that causes harm. The harmed party is entitled to compensation.

There are two types of torts:

- *Unintentional torts* are accidents or mistakes that cause harm.
- *Intentional torts* are deliberate acts that are intended to do harm.

The medical assistant's action was an unintentional tort. About 90 percent of lawsuits against physicians fall into this category.

When a lawsuit claims an unintentional tort, it means that the accuser, called the **plaintiff,** believes a mistake was made.

However, the plaintiff also believes that the accused party, called the **defendant,** did not intend for the mistake to occur.

UNINTENTIONAL TORTS

Most unintentional torts involve **negligence.** Negligence is failure to take reasonable steps to prevent harm. In general, it means that one of two things took place:

- The provider did something that a reasonable health care provider would not have done.
- The provider *failed* to do something that a reasonable health care provider *would* have done.

There are three kinds of malpractice:

- *malfeasance*—wrongful or unlawful treatment
- *misfeasance*—lawful treatment performed incorrectly
- *nonfeasance*—treatment delayed or not attempted.

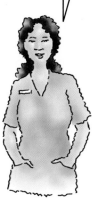

In a health care setting, negligence is often called <u>malpractice.</u>

Standard of Care

In many malpractice cases, the standard of care is an important issue. The **standard of care** is what most professionals with the same type of training would do in a particular situation. Each side in a lawsuit may call witnesses to state what the proper standard of care was in that situation.

Standards of care aren't the same for all levels of professionals. For example, a nurse wouldn't be expected to provide the same care as a physician. A medical assistant wouldn't be held to the same standard of care as a nurse.

This is one reason why medical assistants must never refer to themselves as a nurse. In a lawsuit, a court could hold the actions of a medical assistant who used that title to a nurse's standard of care.

"The Thing Speaks for Itself"

In some cases, the plaintiff's lawyer may apply a principle of law known as **res ipsa loquitur.** This Latin term means "the thing speaks for itself." In other words, it's clear that the defendant's negligence caused the injury. An example might be a fracture that occurred when the patient fell from an examining table.

INTENTIONAL TORTS

An intentional tort is a deliberate violation of another person's legal rights. Intentional torts can also be crimes. Assault and battery, for example, are criminal acts as well as torts.

Secrets for Success   **LEARN WORD PARTS: PREFIXES**

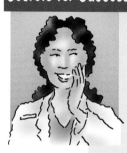

Words are made up of different parts. The main part of the word is called the *root*. A *prefix* can be added to the beginning of the word to change the meaning. Here are some common prefixes you might come across in medical terms.

- *bi-* means *two*
- *mis-* means *wrong*
- *mal-* means *bad*
- *multi-* means *many*
- *mono-* means *one*
- *non-* means *not*
- *pre-* means *before*
- *tri-* means *three*

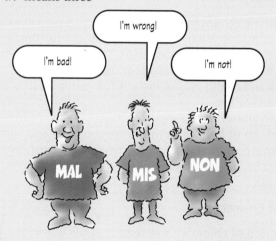

Word to the Wise   **res ipsa loquitur**
(rez IP-suh LOK-wee-toor)

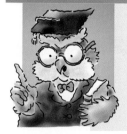

Latin term that means "the thing speaks for itself"; this is a legal term that is used when it's clear that the defendant's negligence caused harm.

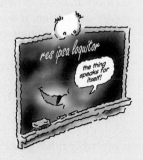

Assault and Battery

Assault is a threat or attempt to touch someone without that person's consent. **Battery** is the actual touching of a person without consent. An example of battery in a health care setting might be giving a patient an injection when she says she does not want one.

Fraud

Fraud is any act that is carried out with the intention of concealing the truth. In the practice of health care, examples include:

- not telling a patient about a treatment's possible side effects
- intentionally raising false hopes for recovery
- filing false insurance claims

Invasion of Privacy

Patients have certain legal rights to privacy. A patient's right to keep information about his or her health and treatment private is known as **patient confidentiality.** It's a term you'll hear often in your work as a medical assistant. You must protect a patient's personal and health information unless giving it out is allowed or required by law.

HIPAA allows you to share a patient's protected information with his or her health insurance company and with all health care providers who are involved in his treatment. In the past, you had to get the patient's permission to do this. Now you do not.

Defamation of Character

Defamation of character is making false or intentionally harmful statements about people that damage their reputations. When these statements are written, it is called **libel.** Speaking such statements is known as **slander.**

Suppose that a patient in your office needs to be referred to a specialist. She tells you that she's heard that Dr. Rogers is a good surgeon. You have heard that Dr. Rogers is an alcoholic. You tell the patient that Dr. Rogers is probably not a good choice because of his

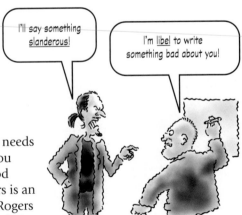

I'll say something slanderous!

I'm libel to write something bad about you!

Legal Brief PERMISSION FORMS

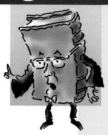

Some offices still have patients sign a permission form, even though the law no longer requires it. However, HIPAA requires that you still must get the patient's permission in other situations. Here are some examples:

- discussing the patient's health information with family members, or even revealing that the office is seeing him
- releasing any health information to the patient's employer
- providing the patient's information to a company to which he's applied for life insurance
- giving the patient's information to any company that is selling a product or service

If you give out information in any of these situations, and the patient has not signed a permission form, he may have a case for invasion of privacy.

drinking. This is slander, and Dr. Rogers could sue you for saying it.

All of the following statements about another person can be defamation of character in certain circumstances:

- saying something that you know is untrue
- saying something harmful with no knowledge whether it is true or false
- saying something with the intention of harming the person's reputation

DEFENSES TO MEDICAL LAWSUITS

Many defenses are available to a health care worker who is being sued.

Medical Records

The best defense a caregiver has is the medical record. Every item in a patient's record is part of a legal document. Juries tend to believe the information that is in the medical record no matter what witnesses at the trial may say or remember. This is because the entries in a patient's chart are a record from the actual time of the event.

The legal implication of the medical record is one reason why what you write in a patient's chart must be timely and readable, as well as thorough and accurate. For example, when you take a patient's medical history, write something like this: "Patient reports no headaches, seizures, or one-sided weakness." It's not enough to write, "Neurological history was negative." This statement provides no specific documentation for the record. Entries in the medical record will refresh the defendant's memory. They also provide evidence of the care the patient received.

Assumption of Risk

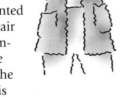

There is a saying in the medical-legal world: "If it's not in the chart, it didn't happen."

Physicians who use the assumption of risk defense will claim that the patient knew the treatment involved risks. However, the patient chose to go ahead with it anyway. In other words, the patient accepted the possibility that things might go wrong. Having a signed consent form in the patient's record can make this defense a strong one.

For example, a patient became bald while she was having chemotherapy treatments for cancer. The patient wanted to sue the physician for causing her hair to fall out. However, hair loss is a common side effect of chemotherapy. She had signed a consent form that said she had been informed of the risks. In this instance, the patient does not have a strong case.

Res Judicata

In some cases, a physician may be able to use a legal principle called **res judicata** as a defense. This is a Latin term that means "the thing has been decided." The legal principle is that once a lawsuit has been settled, the losing party cannot sue the winner. For example, suppose a physician sues a patient for not paying his bill, and the court orders the patient to pay. The patient cannot then sue the physician for malpractice.

Statute of Limitations

Every state has a law that limits the length of time a patient has to file a suit against a health care provider. This legal time limit is called the **statute of limitations.** After that time, the

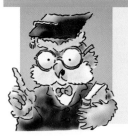

Word to the Wise

res judicata (rez YOO-dee-KAH-tuh)

Latin term that means "the thing has been decided"; this legal term means that once the lawsuit has been settled between the two parties, the losing party cannot sue the winner.

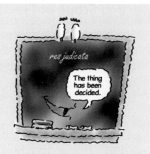

person loses the right to sue. Generally, the statute of limitations expires one to three years after the alleged wrongdoing took place. But some states measure the time from the date the patient *discovers* that wrongdoing may have occurred.

State laws vary greatly when the alleged wrongdoing involves a minor. The statute of limitations might not even begin until the patient becomes an adult and then extend two or three years from that date. Some states also have longer statutes of limitations if alleged wrongdoing may have caused a patient's death.

DEFENSE FOR THE MEDICAL ASSISTANT

Respondeat superior is a legal principle that is also known as the law of agency. The term itself means "let the master answer." This legal principle makes physicians legally responsible for the actions of their employees. However, some very important conditions apply.

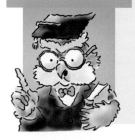

Word to the Wise

respondeat superior (ray-SPON-day-aht soo-PEH-ree-ore)

Latin for "let the master answer"; this legal term means the employer, in this case a physician, is responsible for the actions of employees in the workplace.

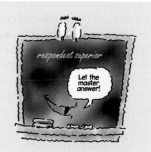

The Law and Scope of Practice

The physician is responsible for your actions only as long as they are within your **scope of practice.** A scope of practice is the range of tasks that a health care provider or some other professional is trained to perform. State law determines the scope of practice for some professions. Your scope of practice will be determined by your training and by the duties your employer assigns to you.

As a new medical assistant, you should guard against stepping outside your scope of practice. If your actions exceed your training or duties, the physician generally isn't responsible for them. If something bad results, you could be sued. The principle of respondeat superior would not protect you in such a case.

Ethics and Health Care

Ethics are guidelines for determining right and wrong. Laws and rules also do this, but they are made and enforced by government. Ethics are set by professional organizations and **peer**

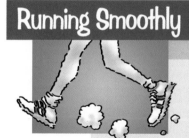

Running Smoothly
ACTING WITHIN YOUR SCOPE OF PRACTICE

What if a patient calls with a medical complaint when the physician is not available?

Mrs. Smith calls the office frequently with minor medical concerns. Today, she's complaining of tingling in her arms. The physician has left for the day, so you tell Mrs. Smith, "Don't worry. Take your medication and call us tomorrow."

That night a blood vessel bursts in Mrs. Smith's brain and she dies. The family sues. The physician says that you weren't authorized to give medical advice over the telephone. You'll be a defendant in the lawsuit because you acted outside your scope of practice.

The proper response is to refer such calls to an office nurse, if one is available. A nurse is trained to recognize what Mrs. Smith's tingling might mean. Medical assistants generally are not. If a nurse isn't available, you should tell such callers to go to an emergency room if they are concerned.

review. Peer review is a process in which a professional's actions are judged by others who work in his or her field. Peer review is very common in health care. It's a major way that health care professionals make sure that standards remain high.

As a medical assistant, you'll encounter issues involving **medical ethics** and possibly **bioethics** as well.

- *Medical ethics* are principles of conduct that govern the behavior of health professionals. They determine proper manners in medical settings, medical customs, and professional courtesy.

- *Bioethics* are moral issues that affect patients' lives. Many of these issues have resulted from advances in modern medicine.

MEDICAL ETHICS FOR MEDICAL ASSISTANTS

As a medical assistant, you will represent the physician in many situations. Your behavior must meet certain ethical standards. You are expected to:

- protect the privacy of patient information
- follow all state and federal laws
- be honest in all your actions

You must always follow ethical standards as you perform your duties. You must ignore your personal feelings of right and

Closer Look   BIOETHICS ISSUES

Advances in technology pose difficult ethical problems in the areas of obstetrics and organ transplantation.

- Obstetrics issues such as when life begins, ownership of fertilized eggs, genetic engineering, and gender selection by parents aren't easily settled.

- As organ transplantation has been perfected, more transplants are being done. Far fewer organs are available than are needed. Every year thousands of patients die who would have been saved by an organ transplant. Deciding who gets available organs sometimes raises ethical issues. So does the fact that many poor countries have become sources of organs, because people sell their body parts to meet basic needs.

wrong if they differ from the ethics of your profession. For example, a medical assistant who opposes abortion must not let his feelings affect how he treats patients seeking abortions. You must show all patients the same kindness and respect. You should never share your personal opinions about medical issues with them.

The Patient Comes First

Your most important responsibility as a medical assistant is to place the patient's best interests first at all times. This may mean that you must set aside your personal value system. On the other hand, you should never be forced to *do* something that violates your value system.

You come first.

Patient Confidentiality

Patient confidentiality is one of the most important ethical principles a medical assistant must observe. You already know that the patient's medical information can't be released without his or her consent, unless it's allowed by law.

In addition, whatever you say to, hear from, or do to a patient is confidential. Patients will reveal some of their innermost thoughts, feelings, and fears. This information is not for public knowledge. Family members, friends, pastors, and others may ask how a patient is doing. Many of these questions are asked with good intentions. However, no information should be released to them without the patient's consent.

Honesty

Honesty is one of the most important qualities for a medical assistant to have. Everyone makes mistakes. How you handle your mistakes shows your ethical standards.

The ability to admit mistakes and take full responsibility for them is the mark of a true professional.

If you make a mistake, such as giving the wrong medication, you must immediately inform your supervisor and the physician. Be honest when speaking to patients about their medical issues.

- Give patients the facts in a clear manner.
- Never offer false expectations or false hope.
- Never minimize or exaggerate the risks of a treatment.

If you don't know the answer to a question, admit that you don't know but say that you will find out. You could also suggest that the patient ask the physician.

AAMA Code of Ethics

The American Association of Medical Assistants (AAMA) is one of the two national organizations that certify medical assistants. It has stated five principles that medical assistants should follow.

1. Provide services with respect for human dignity.
2. Respect patient confidentiality, except when information is required by law.
3. Uphold the honor and high principles set forth by the AAMA.
4. Continually improve knowledge and skills for the benefit of patients and the health care team.
5. Take part in community services and activities that promote good health and welfare to the general public.

WITHHOLDING OR WITHDRAWING TREATMENT

Physicians have a professional and ethical duty to protect life and relieve suffering. Sometimes this duty conflicts with a patient's wishes. Patients have the right to refuse treatments that will sustain their lives. They also have the right to discontinue such treatments.

- *Withholding treatment* means that certain medical treatments will not be started.

- *Withdrawing treatment* means stopping a treatment that has already begun.

Closer Look   **THE MEDICAL ASSISTANT'S CREED**

The AAMA has also written a creed for medical assistants. This pledge is generally recited as a group during graduation or pinning ceremonies.
"I believe in the principles and purposes of the profession of medical assisting.
I endeavor to be more effective.
I aspire to render greater service.
I protect the confidence entrusted to me.
I am dedicated to the care and well-being of all people.
I am loyal to my employer.
I am true to the ethics of my profession.
I am strengthened by compassion, courage, and faith."

Congress passed the Self-Determination Act in 1991. This law gives people who enter the hospital the right to make decisions about their care when they're admitted. These decisions are known as advance directives.

An **advance directive** is a statement of a person's wishes for treatment if a life-threatening event occurs and the patient isn't able to communicate. Advance directives may include specific guidance, such as the following:

- if CPR (Cardiopulmonary Resuscitation) should be started in an attempt to revive the patient
- if a ventilator should be used to help the patient breathe
- if a feeding tube should be inserted to provide nourishment

Merely completing an advance directive does not ensure it will be carried out. The patient also needs to make family members aware of his or her wishes. The patient's next of kin should keep a copy of the advance directive. A clearly marked copy should also be kept in the patient's medical office chart.

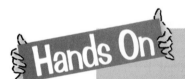

RELEASING MEDICAL RECORDS   2-1

Use these guidelines to ensure that you follow the laws and procedures that protect patient confidentiality.

1. First, have the patient, or the patient's legal guardian, authorize the release of the patient's records in writing.
   - One exception is when providing the information is allowed or required by law.
   - Another exception is when a court orders the records to be released.
2. When releasing a medical record, provide a copy only. Never release the original record unless it is required by a court of law. (See number 7 below.)
3. Determine what part of the record to release. The law requires that only information related to the reason for the request may be released.
   - When copying records, place a piece of blank white paper over any information not authorized for release.

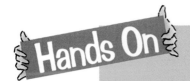

**RELEASING MEDICAL
RECORDS (*continued*)**

- Never permanently white-out information in the original record.
- Never reveal what the blank areas are on a copy of a record.

4. Be sure that you don't release information about mental health conditions or treatment for drug or alcohol abuse (except as required by law) unless the patient gives written permission to do so.

5. *Never* release information over the phone. You have no way of knowing for sure if the person calling is authorized to have the information.

6. When patients request copies of their own records, ask the physician about what parts of the record to copy. In most cases, minors cannot get copies of their medical records unless a parent or guardian has signed a consent form.

7. Only release an original record when it is ordered by a court of law. Otherwise, provide a copy.
   - The physician should ask the judge to sign a form taking temporary charge of the record. The form should be filed in the medical office until the court is finished with the record.
   - As soon as it is known that a record will be part of a court case, it should be kept in a locked cabinet.
   - An office employee should take the record to court each day and return it to the medical office at the end of the day.

8. If the laws in your state permit, and if the physician instructs you to do so, the office may charge a reasonable fee for copying a record that is requested by someone other than the patient.
   - The American Medical Association (AMA) recommends that the fee be no more than $1 per page, with a maximum charge of $100.
   - If fewer than 10 pages are copied, the office may wish to charge as much as $10 to cover the copying, postage, and other expenses.

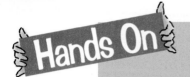

PRESCRIPTION PAD SAFETY PROCEDURES

2-2

1. Keep only one prescription pad in a locked cabinet in the examining room. All other pads should be locked away somewhere else.

2. Keep only a small supply of pads on hand. It's better to reorder on a regular basis than to risk having a large number stolen.

3. Keep track of the number of pads in the office. If a theft occurs, you'll be able to tell police exactly how many are missing.

4. Report prescription pad theft to the police and alert local pharmacies. If the theft involves controlled substance pads, you must also notify the DEA.

5. *Never* leave prescription pads unattended. It takes only seconds for someone to steal a pad or tear off blank prescription forms from it.

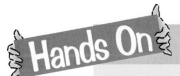

AVOIDING LAWSUITS

2-3

You can take several steps to help you and your employer avoid lawsuits.

1. Keep medical records neat and organized. Always write and sign legibly.

2. Be informed about new laws and medical technology.

3. Keep your CPR and first aid certifications current.

4. Never give out any patient information over the phone unless you know who the caller is and you have the patient's consent.

5. Keep the office neat and clean. Perform safety checks regularly.

6. Make sure that children's toys are clean and in good condition to avoid injuries.

7. Limit waiting time for patients.

8. If an emergency will cause a long wait, inform the patients of the delay in a timely and professional manner.

9. Practice good public relations. Always be polite, smile, and show that you truly care about patients and their families.

10. Make sure your job description is in written form and always perform within its guidelines.

11. Become a CMA or RMA.

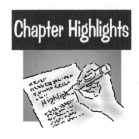

Chapter Highlights

- The fields of medicine and law share an interest in the health and rights of medical patients.

- Lawsuits for malpractice have become more common. Being aware of and following legal requirements will help avoid lawsuits and other legal problems. Good patient-relations practices also help to avoid lawsuits.

- The physician-patient relationship is a legal contract in which each party has rights and responsibilities. Informed consent and the privacy of medical information are important patient rights.

- Many laws and rules apply to health care. Some require reporting confidential patient information. Others regulate working in health care, health care practices and procedures, and the work environment.

- Lawsuits can result from harmful acts by health care workers or because they failed to perform necessary acts. Health care workers can be sued whether their actions or inactions were accidental or intentional.

- Medical records are among the best defenses against lawsuits. Medical assistants can help protect against lawsuits by careful and thorough charting.

- Medical assistants can be sued in certain circumstances. They can protect themselves by not acting in ways that exceed their training or the duties assigned by their employer.

- Medical ethics and bioethics can involve complicated issues that have no easy answers. A medical assistant's first responsibility is always to act with the patient's rights and best interests in mind.

- Ethical standards for medical assistants include putting the patient first, protecting patient privacy, always acting honestly, and following the AAMA code of ethics.

Chapter 3

OPERATIONAL FUNCTIONS

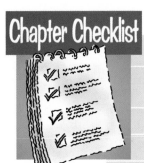

Chapter Checklist

- Identify the basic parts of a computer
- Perform routine maintenance of administrative and clinical equipment
- Describe types of administrative software for a medical office
- Utilize computer software to maintain office systems
- Discuss the ethics of computer access
- Explain the basics of conducting searches on the Internet
- Explain how quality improvement and risk management work together to improve patient care and employee needs
- Summarize the guidelines for completing incident reports
- Use methods of quality control
- Perform an inventory of supplies and equipment

To be successful, a medical office must function efficiently and effectively. As a medical assistant, you'll have an important role in making sure the office runs smoothly. Appointment schedules must be made and followed. Patient charts and other records must be maintained accurately. Systems must be in place to ensure that the office has a steady flow of income and that it provides high-quality care. Equipment must be kept in good working order and needed supplies must be on hand at all times. In the modern medical office, many of these tasks involve using the office's computers.

The Office Computer System

Computers play a major role in the operation of a medical office. You'll use them every day. Here are just a few of the ways you might do so:

- preparing letters and memos
- scheduling appointments for patients
- processing claims with patients' insurance companies
- posting charges and payments to patients' accounts
- checking on lab results for the physician
- helping the physician prescribe medications

As you can see, being a medical assistant requires good computer skills. To strengthen these skills, let's review some basics about computers.

The computers in your office have two main systems—the hardware system and the software system. **Hardware** is the actual machinery or equipment. **Software** is the electronic "instructions" that tell the hardware what to do. Each set of instructions is called a **program** or an **application.** *Application* is the "techie" term for *program.* They mean the same thing.

A computer's software includes many programs. Each lets you use the computer to perform a specific task, such as scheduling appointments, writing a letter, and so on. You'll read more about this later.

COMPUTER HARDWARE

Your computer's hardware includes several key pieces of equipment. Here's a list of the most important ones.

1. *Central Processing Unit (CPU).* Think of this as the "brain" of the computer. The CPU, or **microprocessor,** carries out instructions sent to it by the software stored on the computer. The CPU tells the computer how to operate a given program.

2. *Hard drive.* This stores the computer's programs and data. Think of the hard drive as the memory of the CPU brain. The capacity of a hard drive is measured in megabytes or gigabytes.

3. *Monitor.* The monitor looks like a television screen. It displays the information sent to it by the CPU. The quality of the image is based on the monitor's DPI (dots per inch) setting. The more DPIs, the clearer the picture. Like TVs, monitors come in various sizes and have controls for adjusting brightness and contrast.

4. *Keyboard.* This is the main way to enter information into the computer. It has keys for each letter, numeral, and punctuation mark. It also has several special function keys. They include Alt, Ctrl, and F1 through F12. Each special function key has a dif-

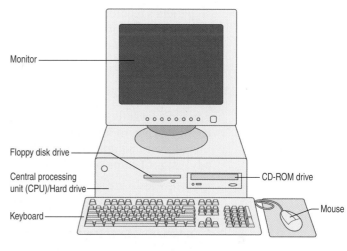

ferent use based on the program being used. For instance, certain keys may do the following:
- search for and replace words
- move or copy blocks of text
- indent or center text
- check spelling and grammar

5. *Mouse.* This device moves the **cursor,** or pointer arrow, on the monitor's display screen.

6. **Modem.** A modem connects the computer to e-mail and the Internet. This connection can be through a phone line, a TV cable, or a digital subscriber line (DSL).

7. *Printer.* The printer transfers information from the computer to paper. Printers work at various speeds. They can print letters, bills, and other documents. In computer talk, this output is called **hard copy.**
- Dot matrix printers are used mainly for printing multicopy insurance forms. Their print quality is usually not good enough for patient instructions or letters.
- Laser printers produce high quality documents. They can be expensive, but they are common in medical offices.
- Ink jet printers often cost less than laser printers. They also produce high quality copies. They can print in color as well as black and white.

8. *Scanner.* This device allows you to put hard copy into the computer. Lab reports can be scanned into a

> The modem can be contained in the computer's hardware, or it can be a separate piece of equipment.

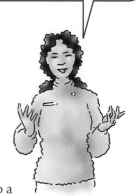

patient's record, for instance. You also could scan patient education information into the computer, change it, and then print copies of the new version.

SAVING FILES

You have several choices for saving the files you create or change on a computer. One option, of course, is to save them to your computer's hard drive. You also can take advantage of some portable storage options.

- Floppy disks are small (3.5-inch) plastic cases that fit into a computer's disk drive. They have very limited storage capacity (about 2 megabytes). Most new computers no longer have disk drives.

- Compact disks (CDs) hold more data than floppy disks, but their capacity is limited to about 700 megabytes. Usually, data saved on them is "read-only." This means the files can't be changed and resaved on the same disk.

- Zip drives plug into your computer and hold what might be described as large floppy disks. Like floppy disks, zip storage is old technology. However, disks for newer zip drives can hold as much as 2 gigabytes of data. (A gigabyte is 1,000 megabytes.)

- Digital video disks (DVDs) use technology much like CDs. However, they hold several times more data— about 5 gigabytes. Files stored on DVDs will be readable for more than 70 years.

- Flash drives (sometimes called jump drives) also plug into your computer. But they are so small that they can fit on a key chain. This makes it easy to move files from computer to computer. Some flash drives can hold 16 gigabytes of data.

- External hard drives are larger storage devices that you can plug into you computer. Like zip drives and flash drives, they come in various amounts of storage capacity. Some external hard drives can hold 600 gigabytes of data.

Your office will likely have procedures for how you should save and store your files. It is important that you follow these procedures carefully so that valuable data won't be lost.

Computer Care

Treat your computer well, just as you would all office equipment. Computers do require special attention, however. Here are some guidelines for taking care of your computer.

- Keep your computer in a cool, dry area out of direct sunlight. Excess heat and humidity can damage its parts.
- Your computer or desk should be on an antistatic mat or carpet. Static electricity can cause memory loss and inaccurate processing of data.
- Keep computers away from magnets.
- Do not eat or drink while working at the computer. If you spill any liquid or crumbs into the keyboard, it might not work properly.
- Plug your computer into a surge protector instead of directly into the electrical outlet. Without surge protection, changes in the office's power supply could damage the computer's parts.
- Your computer should have a battery backup power source. This will prevent the loss of data if there's a power failure. If you move a computer, lock the hard drive. This helps protect its CPU from damage.

The Hands On procedure about computer care on page 123 gives you more procedures for taking care of a computer.

Handhelds

Many physicians use handheld computers. This type of computer is also known as a personal digital assistant (PDA). Information is entered with a stylus, a pointed device that's shaped like a pen, or on a small keyboard. PDAs also can be attached to a regular-size computer keyboard.

The physician can use a PDA to send information to your desktop computer and receive information from it. For instance, you could send the physician's PDA a note from your computer that a patient called the office and asked the physician to call her back. But keep in mind that not all physicians will want to communicate this way. Always check with the physician before passing along important messages in a new way.

PDAs can send information to each other. They also can use a cell phone to connect to the Internet. Here are some other things a physician can do with a PDA:

- access patients' charts
- view financial data
- access medical and pharmacy information
- view procedures they may not do very often

There are many computer software programs available for a PDA. There are programs that include information from medical reference books and foreign language dictionaries that can be stored in this handheld computer.

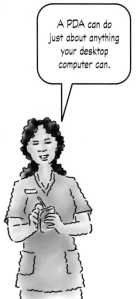

A PDA can do just about anything your desktop computer can.

Computer Networks

If your office has just two or three computers, each one may be separate from the others. Offices with more computers may have them connected in an **intranet.** This is a private data-sharing network of computers. Usually, only people using the office computers can get on the network. But some intranets can be accessed from home computers, too.

THE INTRANET

An intranet gives you quick access to information including:

- policy and procedure manuals
- common office forms
- phone lists
- staff schedules
- office newsletters or job postings
- agendas for upcoming meetings
- local hospital information
- support for video conferencing
- links to special sites on the Internet

OFFICE SOFTWARE

Many software programs are useful in a medical office. Some help with running the office. Other programs, such as clinical software, directly aid the practice of medicine. The software you'll use will depend on several factors. These include:

- the office's health care specialty
- your duties in the office
- software used by any hospital associated with the office

Let's look at some basic types of administrative applications. These are programs for the office's daily business operations.

Scheduling

Scheduling patients by computer is more efficient than using a paper appointment book. User-friendly scheduling software helps you find open appointment times more quickly. It also lets you make changes more easily. Good scheduling software should perform the following functions:

- offer an unlimited comment area near the patient's name; this lets you add special reminder notes for the appointment—for instance, "Patient wants a pregnancy test."

- keep a list of patients who want to move their appointments if a more suitable one becomes available.

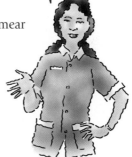

Some software allows patients to schedule their own appointments using the Internet. This convenience can result in fewer calls to the office and happier patients.

- print notices to remind patients that they need to make appointments; for example, the program could be set to alert patients who regularly have an annual Pap smear that it's time to make an appointment.

Some appointment software can connect to the appointment software of other offices. This is useful if a patient needs to be seen by a health care provider in another office. You can make the patient an appointment with the other provider without having to call his or her office.

Tracking

Some software helps the office run more efficiently by tracking the flow of patients. Here are just of few of the things this software can do.

- show which days of the week tend to be busiest or the slowest and which have the most cancelled appointments; this information can help schedule staff more efficiently.

- track the activity of providers; for example, one physician may average 45 minutes per patient. Another may average

30 minutes. This kind of information can help you in scheduling appointments.

- track the time patients wait in the reception area or an examination room; long waiting times can show a need for better procedures or more staff.

Insurance

Software programs send claims via the computer's modem or cable lines to the patient's health insurance company. Filing claims this way results in faster payment. It also allows you to track the progress of claims better and identify any problems that could cause a delay in payment.

Other insurance programs perform other functions, such as:

- allow you to check that the patient is eligible for coverage
- provide preapproval of certain procedures and hospital admissions (You'll read about this in Chapters 4 and 8.)
- help you properly code health care services when submitting claims for insurance (You'll read about coding in Chapter 7.)

Federal law now requires that nearly all insurance claims be submitted by computer.

Financial

A large number of programs can help you with the office's finances. Some of them track accounts receivable (money that's owed to the office) and accounts payable (money the office owes to others). Other programs will figure what each patient owes and prepare the bills the office mails out each month. Here are some examples of even more financial software.

- Some programs alert you when a patient's account is seriously past due. They even have form letters that you can send to demand payment. (Chapter 6 gives you more information about collecting overdue accounts.)
- Some software accepts and automatically deposits insurance payments directly in the

Always check a patient's account before having the computer prepare a collection letter. Collection letters should be sent only when necessary.

office's bank account. This saves you from having to handle, record, process, and deposit these payments yourself.

- Special software will let the office take payments by credit card. Some patients will want to pay what they owe this way. Every medical office should be able to accept payments charged to the four major credit cards—American Express, Discover Card, Master-Card, and Visa.

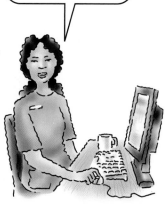

Medical software is not just for office administration. Some programs have valuable clinical uses.

Other Software

A medical office needs a word processing system to run effectively. This is the software that lets you write letters, address envelopes, and prepare other kinds of documents.

Software programs are also available that manage the office payroll and employees' personnel records.

Some programs document that your office is complying with HIPAA—the Health Insurance Portability and Accountability Act. This federal law requires health care providers to follow certain rules about patients' privacy.

Closer Look   CLINICAL SOFTWARE

Software assists the delivery of health care, too. Here are just three examples of what clinical software can do.

- Some programs insert lab reports directly into a patient's chart. This eliminates errors that can occur when a person records the results in the chart. Most of these programs also alert the physician when a new report has been received.

- Programs help physicians write prescriptions. This eliminates errors from poor handwriting. Some programs warn the physician if the prescription is not correct for the patient's medical condition or with other drugs the patient is taking.

- With some programs, physicians can view x-rays and other tests on the computer. The physician does not have to wait for the written report. She can judge the test results herself.

COMPUTER ETHICS

As you can see, computers are a must in all medical offices. They save time and make operations more efficient. They also make it much easier to gather and provide information. But a computer's usefulness also has a potential for abuse. Misuse can lead to invasion of patients' privacy and other unethical behavior.

Here are some tips for using the office computers. If you follow these guidelines, your computer use will remain ethical and legal.

- Never give out the password you use to log on to the computer or to access a certain program or data. Each employee should have his or her own password.
- Never use another person's password to get patient information. If you're authorized to see this information, ask for a password of your own.
- If you can access a lab's computer to get test results, don't obtain results on people who are not office patients. For example, suppose that your son had a test at another doctor's office that was sent to a lab to which you have access. You shouldn't look up his test results, even though he's your son.
- Never leave a patient's information displayed on the monitor and walk away from a computer. Close the file before leaving your computer.
- Don't use the office computer to surf the Internet for personal reasons. This isn't appropriate behavior at work.
- Never load any software into your office computer unless you have permission. Doing this could cause conflicts with the office software as well as other problems.

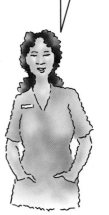

Instant messaging software doesn't belong in the workplace. Limit its use to your personal time.

E-MAIL GUIDELINES

Here are some guidelines for using your office computer's e-mail program.

- Don't read e-mails for the physician or other staff that are sent to the office's general e-mail address. Each staff member should have his or her own office e-mail address. You should forward the e-mail to that person's address.
- It's never appropriate to receive personal mail at your office e-mail address. It's also not appropriate to access your personal e-mail while at work.
- Don't send sensitive patient information by e-mail unless you're sure the person receiving the e-mail is the only one who can access it.

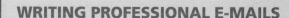

Secrets for Success   WRITING PROFESSIONAL E-MAILS

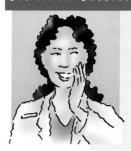

Use these tips to maintain a professional tone in your e-mail messages:

- Always check your spelling, grammar, and punctuation before you send any e-mails. Poor grammar or incorrect spelling can take away from your message.

- Keep messages short and to the point. Remember, you are not entertaining the reader. You are communicating information to him or her.

- Avoid colored fonts or cute figures in your e-mails. Imagine your e-mail as a typewritten business letter.

- Always fill in the subject line. Give the reader a sense of what your e-mail is about. For example, "Staff meeting tomorrow," tells your reader the essence of the message.

- Never send an e-mail to the physician about an emergency situation. Call or page the physician instead.

Closer Look   PASSWORDS

Many of the things you'll do on the computer will require a password. Here are some guidelines for creating and protecting the passwords you choose.

- Combine letters and numbers in each password you create.

- Avoid using your name, initials, birth date, phone number, and the word *password* as passwords.

- Do not tape your password on your computer or leave it in your desk.

- Change your password from time to time or if you suspect that someone else knows what it is.

Internet Basics

Your office probably can connect to the Internet. Most medical offices can. The Internet can be helpful to the office in a number of ways.

CONNECTING TO THE NET

The first thing your office needs to use the Internet is an Internet service provider (ISP). This is a company that connects your computer to the Internet. America Online, Earthlink, and Road-runner are three well-known national ISPs. But hundreds of such companies exist.

Get Connected!

ISPs can connect your computer to the Internet in one of four ways.

- *Dial-up service.* This connection is through a standard telephone line. It's the cheapest and the slowest way to connect.
- *Cable Internet.* This method uses the cable system operated by a cable television company. It's more expensive than dial-up service. But it's also much faster.
- *DSL connection.* DSL stands for digital subscriber line. It uses a special telephone line designed especially for Internet connections. It is also more expensive and faster than a dial-up connection.
- *Satellite connection.* This method uses TV satellite dishes to connect to the Internet.

> If you're going to be downloading large files from the Internet, you should have a broadband connection for speed and efficiency.

DSL, cable, and satellite connections are known as high-speed or broadband connections. They have become more popular as the kinds and size of files on the Internet have increased. Video files, for example, can be huge. You might have to stay online for hours to download a video if you're using dial-up service.

Just Browsing, Thank You

Another thing you'll need to connect to the Internet is a web browser. This is software on your computer that communicates with the Internet. Two common examples are Internet Explorer and Netscape. Many computers come with Internet Explorer already installed on them.

Let's Go Surfing!

Once you're online, the process of searching the Internet is called **surfing.** Often, a **search engine** can help you find the information you need. A search engine is a program on the Internet that searches millions of Internet sites for the desired information. Some of the more popular search engines are:

- AltaVista
- Dogpile
- Excite
- Google
- Lycos
- Yahoo

Each of these search engines has different features. AltaVista, for example, lets you translate information from other languages into English. Dogpile combines several other search engines with its own.

Your Search Results

When you surf the Internet, there's one important thing you need to keep in mind—anyone can put anything on the Internet. Information found on websites may not be accurate or even truthful.

Because information you get from the Internet may affect patient care, you must be sure it's accurate. One way to do this is to look for the HON seal on the Internet site. *HON* stands for Health on the Net Foundation. HON is a private nonprofit organization. It's dedicated to improving the quality of medical information on the Internet. Its seal means that the site's information meets HON's standards for reliability.

Of course, plenty of other sites on the Internet provide accurate medical information, too. For example, government sites are good sources of information. So are the sites of medical journals and professional medical organizations.

The HON seal is a good starting point, however. The table *Basic Medical Sources on the Internet* gives you some other sites to use as well. You may want to **bookmark** these sites on your web browser. The Running Smoothly box on page 112 gives you clues about the types of sites to avoid.

Each physician in your office will have a specialty. Know the Internet addresses of journals and professional organizations for that specialty. Suppose you work for a neurologist, for instance. You'd want to bookmark the address of the American Academy of Neurology (www.aan.com).

> Bookmarking a website lets you go directly to it without using a search engine.

Basic Medical Sources on the Internet

Site	Internet Address	Description
American Medical Association (AMA)	www.ama-assn.org	Contains information on many subjects related to the practice of medicine
Centers for Disease Control (CDC)	www.cdc.gov	Offers information on a variety of health care topics
Cinhal Information Systems	www.cinhal.com	Includes articles for nurses and other allied health care professionals
NLM Gateway	gateway.nlm.nih.gov	Connects users with 18 different collections of medical information
PubMed Central	pubmedcentral.nih.gov	Contains thousands of articles on many health care subjects from different journals

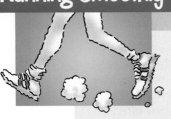

Running Smoothly

MEDICAL INFORMATION ON THE NET

What if a physician asks you to find information about a medical topic on the Internet?

Let's say the physician asks you to find some information on the Internet about heart disease. This information will be used in a patient brochure the office is creating. You entered the term *heart disease* into your search engine. It returned 627,000 web pages on this topic. You want to be sure that information you pick for the brochure is safe to use.

Here are some hints to help you identify which Internet medical information to avoid.

- Stay away from sites that advertise they've cured a disease or that the cure can only be found on that site.

- Beware of terms such as miracle and breakthrough. For instance, a site that calls its vitamin cure for heart disease a "miracle in a bottle" may not contain reliable information.

- Use caution with sites that offer the same treatment for a whole list of diseases.

- If a site suggests that the government or physicians are hiding the truth about a disease or a cure, do not use its information.

- Be careful of any information that's connected to a claim of a secret formula or an ancient remedy.

The Internet and Insurance

The world of health insurance can seem like an endless maze of regulations. The Internet can help you sort through some of this information. Here are a few ways how.

- A patient's insurance card usually lists the Internet address of the insurance company. Many times its website can tell you what kind of coverage the patient has.

- If the physician wants to send a patient for care elsewhere, the patient's insurance company's website often lists places the company prefers provide the treatment.

- The government's Medicare site (www.medicare.gov) provides information about Medicare programs and answers many frequently asked questions.

PATIENT EDUCATION AND THE NET

Some patients will be skilled at using the Internet. They'll be able to find a lot of information about their medical problem, possible treatments, and medications.

The guidelines in the Running Smoothly box on page 112 also apply to patients using the Internet. Patients may turn to the Internet when they feel confused or hopeless about their disease.

You can't stop them, of course, or limit the information they'll find. All you can do is try to teach these patients how to identify reliable and dangerous medical information on the Net.

Some physicians print lists of recommended Internet sites for certain kinds of medical information. This is a good educational tool. The Closer Look feature on page 114 provides some good general patient education sites.

Drugs on the Net

Increasing numbers of people are buying prescription drugs on the Internet. Medication often costs less online than it does at local pharmacies.

If you know patients buy drugs online, you should tell the physician if they take any of these medications:

- Accutane (isotretinion)
- Actiq (fentanyl citrate)
- Clozaril (clozapine)
- Lotronex (alosetron hydrochloride)
- Mifeprex (mifepristone or RU-486)

Closer Look   PATIENT EDUCATION SITES

Here are some Internet sites that offer good health care information to the public.

- American Dental Association: www.ada.org/public/index.asp
- American Sleep Apnea Association: www.sleepapnea.org
- consumer health information: www.health.nih.gov
- health information for seniors: www.nihseniorhealth.gov
- MedlinePlus: www.medlineplus.gov
- *Merck Manual:* www.merckhomeedition.com
- National Attention Deficit Disorder Association: www.add.org
- smoking cessation: www.QuitNet.org
- sources for children with cancer: www.cancersourcekids.com
- travel health: www.cdc.gov/travel

- Thalomid (thalidomide)
- Tikosyn (dofetilide)
- Tracleer (bosentan)

The U.S. Food and Drug Administration (FDA) cautions against buying these drugs on the Internet. People can harm themselves if these drugs are not prescribed correctly. People who are taking them must be watched closely by a physician.

Financial Help on the Net

Sometimes, patients who are having trouble paying for their prescriptions can find help on the Internet. If you know of such a patient, here are some ways you can assist.

- Tell the patient to visit the home page of the company that makes the drug—for example, www.Pfizer.com.

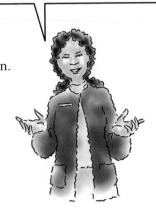

Tell the physician about any patient taking drugs that were prescribed on an Internet site. Even drugs bought online should be prescribed by someone who has seen the patient in person.

Closer Look · COMPUTER SECURITY

The Internet connects you to computers around the world. This can expose the office computer system to a number of dangers. Here are some dangers and some guidelines to keep your computer safe and working well.

1. *Cookies*. These are tiny files that many sites will leave in your hard drive.
   - Some cookies track what you do on the Internet and report it to the site.
   - You can block cookies by setting limits on them on your web browser.

2. *Unsecure information*. Information you fill out on a site might be seen by unauthorized people.
   - Never provide private information to a site that does not have a secure sockets layer (SSL).
   - The SSL scrambles information as it leaves your computer and unscrambles it when it reaches the site.
   - A tiny picture of a lock in your browser's status bar shows if a site is secure.

3. *Viruses*. These can invade your computer and destroy your files and software. They are a major security problem.
   - Never download information, screensavers, or other programs onto your computer from suspicious sites.
   - Only open attachments to e-mail that are sent by known sources. Attachments from unknown sources could contain viruses.
   - Make sure your computer is equipped with virus protection software. Use the updating service that most antivirus programs offer.

4. *Firewalls*. These are computer programs or devices that prevent unauthorized users from accessing private information on your computer's network through the Internet.
   - Firewalls are used to prevent people from gaining entry to private computer networks from outside the network.
   - A firewall builds a list of acceptable websites based on your past use of the computer. Attempts to access sites not on the list are denied.
   - Some firewalls limit the type or content of files your computer can receive.

- Another site to suggest is www.needymeds.com.
- Patients on Medicare can find help at www.medicare.gov/prescription/home.asp.
- Physicians can find help for patients at www.Rxhope.com.

Quality Improvement

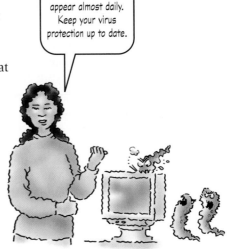

New computer viruses appear almost daily. Keep your virus protection up to date.

Quality Improvement, or QI, is an effort to improve every part of an organization. In health care, QI's main goal is to provide services that meet and exceed patients' needs. Many medical providers are required by law to have QI programs.

QI IN MEDICAL OFFICES

QI programs exist in medical offices mainly because two federal agencies require them.

- The Occupational Safety and Health Administration (OSHA) requires QI programs to protect employees and patients. You read about some OSHA requirements in Chapter 2. You'll learn more about them in your clinical training.
- The Centers for Medicare & Medicaid Services (CMS) requires providers who treat patients covered by Medicare and Medicaid to have QI programs.

Here are some of the ways QI programs can benefit health care organizations.

- identify delays and failures in the delivery system for care
- improve service to patients and their families
- encourage teamwork within the organization
- increase efficiency and productivity
- increase employee morale
- improve patient satisfaction and outcomes

Outcomes are the final results of the care patients receive. Here's an example. A patient arrives in the office with a cut on her leg. The cut is sutured. Six days later the patient returns to have the sutures removed. The wound healed with no complications. This patient's outcome was acceptable.

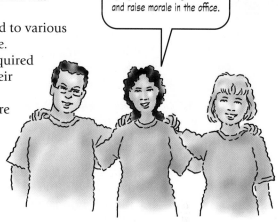

QI programs encourage teamwork and raise morale in the office.

Patient outcomes are reported to various agencies that oversee health care. Currently, only hospitals are required to produce "report cards" on their patient outcomes. But pressure is building in Congress to require all health care providers to do so.

Patients can view report cards on various sites on the Internet. They can use this information to help them select a provider whose services best meet their needs.

MINDING YOUR P'S AND QI'S

The CMS is a division of the U.S. Department of Health and Human Services (HHS). HHS and CMS monitor two federal laws that you first read about in Chapter 2—the Clinical Laboratory Improvement Amendments (CLIA) and the Health Insurance Portability and Accountability Act (HIPAA). Both laws are related to QI because they set standards in many areas of health care. Some of these standards will affect what you do as a medical assistant.

CLIA

Congress passed the Clinical Laboratory Improvement Amendments in 1988. The standards they set improved accuracy in lab test results. Before CLIA, some lab tests, such as Pap smears, were notoriously inaccurate. Patients died as a result.

CLIA set three levels of complexity for lab tests:

- low complexity
- moderate complexity
- high complexity

HHS approves clinical laboratories and physician office labs (POLs) to perform tests at one of these levels. Most POLs can perform only low or moderate complexity tests. Here are some of the tests a POL can perform.

Legal Brief — QUALITY IMPROVEMENT AND HIPAA

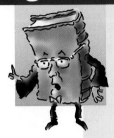

HIPAA was passed to:

- set standards for the security and privacy of patients' health information; these standards are covered in detail in other chapters of this book.
- set standards for submitting claims to patients' health insurers; you'll read about these standards in Chapter 8.

As with CLIA, medical offices need to have QI programs in place to make sure HIPAA standards are being met. For example, HIPAA requires that each medical office have a privacy officer. This person is responsible for seeing that patients' information is handled in the ways HIPAA requires.

- *Low complexity tests:* urine dipsticks, fecal occult blood packets, urine pregnancy tests, ovulation kits, centrifuged microhematocrits, and certain blood glucose tests
- *Moderate complexity tests:* white blood cell counts, Gram staining, packaged rapid strep test, and automated cholesterol testing

All labs must have a QI program to identify and correct testing problems.

Risk Management

Risk management is the process of identifying problems before they cause injury to patients or staff. Potential problems are directly related to risk factors. A risk factor is anything that could be a safety concern. A few typical risk factors in a medical office include:

- poor lighting
- frayed wires on electrical instruments or machines
- improper disposal of needles
- poor procedures for identifying patients

The risk factors just listed could result in these problems:

- patients falling
- electric shock

- needlesticks of employees
- treatment mistakes

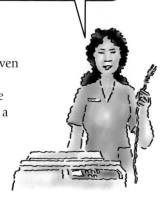

Always be on the lookout for equipment that needs to be fixed or replaced. A frayed wire on this plug is a risk factor that could result in electric shock.

RISK FACTORS

One way to find risk factors in your office is to look for trends in the office's **incident reports.** These are written accounts of negative events experienced by patients, visitors, or staff. Incident reports should be completed for even minor negative events.

If you're involved in or witness a negative event, you'll be expected to file an incident report. Your office probably has a standard form for incident reports that you would fill out. Here's what usually happens next.

- A supervisor reviews the report for completeness and accuracy and sends it on.
- The report will be given to the office manager or the physician. (In a hospital, it would go to the risk manager.)
- The physician may add comments to the report. This will depend on the type of event and the office's policy. If the event involved a patient, the physician will probably assess the patient and record the findings on the report.

Incident Reports

Bad things can happen, even in the safest offices. Sometimes, they result from human errors. Other times, their causes are unknown or unavoidable.

For instance, if you give a patient the wrong medication, that's a human error. You must make an incident report. Now, suppose you gave the patient the correct medication and he had an allergic reaction to it. You still must complete an incident report, even though there was no human error. That's an example of an unavoidable event.

A good rule to follow is, "When in doubt, complete an incident report."

Here are some events that always require an incident report.

- all medication errors
- any fall by a patient, employee, or visitor
- drawing blood from the wrong patient
- incorrect labeling of blood tubes or other lab specimens
- accidental needlesticks of employees
- workers' compensation injuries (work related injuries)

Closer Look — INCIDENT REPORT MYTHS

Many health care professionals try to avoid completing incident reports because of various myths about them. Here are some of these myths and the facts in each case.

- *Myth:* If I complete an incident report, I'll get fired.

Fact: Your employer needs to have a record of negative events. You're more likely to be fired for failing to complete one.

- *Myth:* Incident reports go into my employee file.

Fact: They are not placed in your file. They're stored separately so they can be used for QI.

- *Myth:* If I complete an incident report, I'm admitting I'm at fault.

Fact: Incident reports do not assign fault. They just record what happened.

What Goes in an Incident Report

Your office will have its own incident report form. The Hands On procedure on page 124 provides guidelines for filling it out. The following information always should be included:

- the name, address, and phone number of the injured person
- the birth date and sex of the injured person
- the date, time, and location of the event
- names and addresses of any witnesses
- a brief description of the event and what was done to deal with it
- any tests or treatments that were performed
- patient examination findings, if any
- the signature and title of the person completing the form
- any other signatures required by office policy

INCIDENT REPORTS AND QI

Groups of incident reports can be studied to look for patterns. Finding patterns in negative events can help identify problem areas. These problems can then be corrected through QI

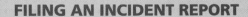

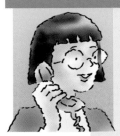

Ask the Professional — **FILING AN INCIDENT REPORT**

Q: *I gave a patient the wrong medication this morning. Fortunately, she didn't have a bad reaction to it. Do I still need to make an incident report? Since she was okay, wouldn't I be better off by not making a record of the error?*

A: You would definitely *not* be better off! If fact, you put yourself at risk if you don't report it. Not filing an incident report could lead to charges of falsifying medical records, tampering with medical records, and not following office policies.

You don't have to say, "I gave the wrong medication." Just state the facts: "X medication was ordered. I gave Y medication." Write whom you told and when, what they advised you to do, and any other important information. If the event results in a lawsuit, having an accurate record of it can help your office's attorney.

programs. Here are examples of how trends found in incident reports can be important to risk management and quality improvement programs.

- *Days of the week when most events happen.* For example, if many events occur on Friday afternoons, staffing for that time period might be evaluated.

- *Most common area for patient falls.* If most falls are in the lobby, a QI program should find out why people are falling there and make the needed changes.

- *Medications that are routinely given incorrectly.* Adding brightly colored warning labels to these drugs might help.

- *The age group most likely to have events.* If incident reports show older patients have the most events, a QI program on caring for this group might be needed for staff.

Office Equipment and Supplies

The average medical office contains a lot of expensive equipment. It also uses a huge amount of supplies. Making sure equipment works correctly and that the office doesn't run out of needed supplies is an important part of quality control.

Broken equipment can keep the office from running smoothly or from running at all. Computer breakdowns could keep you from scheduling appointments, for instance, or from sending out monthly bills. You also wouldn't want to turn away a patient because a piece of clinical equipment wasn't working right.

Service Contracts

A service contract is an arrangement with a company to care for office equipment. For a yearly fee, the company will inspect and service certain equipment, such as a photocopier or an EKG machine. One of your duties may be to keep track of these contracts and make sure that equipment is serviced regularly.

Routine Care of Equipment

Another of your duties may be to make regular checks of clinical equipment to be sure it's working correctly. Your office's QI program may have a schedule that tells how often each type of equipment should be checked.

Checking the accuracy of a blood glucose meter is one example of this task. This responsibility is commonly given to a medical assistant. Medical assistants also may have to check other lab equipment to help the office meet CLIA requirements. Specifically, CLIA requires:

- a system to assure that each piece of lab equipment is producing accurate results on lab tests
- a log for each piece of equipment that shows each time its accuracy was checked and the results of the check

If federal inspectors visit your office lab, they will want to see these records.

Equipment Inventories. You may need to keep track of the office's machines as well as of their performance and accuracy. To run smoothly, every business needs to know what pieces of equipment it has and how many. This list of the number of each item is called an **inventory.**

It's important to have an inventory of equipment in case of a theft, a fire, or some other damage to the office. The Hands On procedure on page 124 gives you the steps for performing an inventory of the office's equipment.

STAYING SUPPLIED

How bad would it be for office operations if you ran out of paper for the printer? Now think about how much worse it could be if you ran out of paper for the EKG machine or sterile pads for dressing wounds.

It's very important that the office is properly supplied. Medical supplies—bottles of sterile water, for instance—often have expiration dates. If too much is on hand, it may expire. And once the sterile water expires, it shouldn't be used. That would cost the office money. On the other hand, you don't want to have so little of something that you might run out of it.

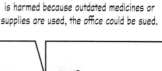

Always discard expired stock. If a patient is harmed because outdated medicines or supplies are used, the office could be sued.

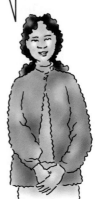

Keeping good records is the key to avoiding both situations. You should make a weekly or monthly inventory of the office's supplies. Comparing these numbers over time will give you an idea of how fast the office uses its stock of each item. This will help you know how much of that item to keep on hand and when it's time to order more.

You may be responsible for the office's entire stock of supplies. Or your job may include tracking only certain types of supplies. In either case, the Hands On procedure on page 126 will guide you in using the spreadsheet software on your computer to perform an inventory of supplies.

Hands On   COMPUTER CARE   `3-1`

Computers are key pieces of administrative equipment. Your office computer should be cleaned regularly. Follow these steps.

1. Remove any CDs or DVDs and close all programs that are running.
2. Shut down the CPU and turn off the monitor.
3. Clean the monitor screen with antistatic wipes. Do not use a regular glass cleaner.
4. Turn the keyboard face down so any loose debris can fall out. Do not shake or tap the keyboard.
5. Use a can of compressed air to blow the remaining dust and particles from under the keyboard's keypads.
6. Use a *damp* (not wet) cloth to clean the underside of the mouse. If the mouse has a roller ball, carefully remove and clean it.
7. Place dust covers over the monitor and keyboard when they are not in use to keep them clean longer.

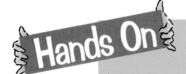

COMPLETING AN INCIDENT REPORT

3-2

Properly completed incident reports are necessary for your office to have an effective quality improvement program. Follow these guidelines when completing an incident report.

1. State only the facts. Don't draw conclusions. For example, if you find a patient on the floor in the waiting area, do not write, "Patient slipped and fell." That draws a conclusion. Instead, write, "Patient found on floor. Patient stated that he fell."

2. Do not leave any blank spaces on the form. Write N/A (for "not applicable") in all areas that do not apply to the situation. This reduces the chance that other comments could be added later.

3. Complete the form in a timely manner. In most cases, an incident report should be written within 24 hours of the event.

4. Write legibly and sign your name. Be sure to include your title.

5. Do not photocopy the report for your own record. Most incident reports contain confidential patient information. Copying them for your own use would be illegal.

6. Do not put a copy of the report in the patient's chart. Record the event in the chart, but do not write that an incident report was completed. This would open the door for a patient's lawyers to subpoena the report if there is a lawsuit.

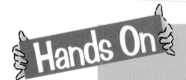

INVENTORY OF OFFICE EQUIPMENT

3-3

A well-run medical office keeps close track of its administrative and clinical equipment. Use these guidelines when preparing an inventory of the equipment in your office.

1. Determine exactly what should be included in the inventory.
   - Should all equipment be included or only equipment that costs more than a set amount of money?

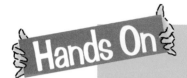

INVENTORY OF OFFICE EQUIPMENT (*continued*)

- Should office furnishings, such as examining tables and waiting room lamps and chairs, be included?

Your supervisor or employer should provide this guidance.

2. Create an inventory sheet for each category of equipment. Categories could be defined by the type of equipment or by its location.
   - There might be a sheet for all computers and a separate sheet for all EKG machines, for example.
   - There might be a separate sheet for each room, on which all the equipment in that room is listed.

3. Prepare columns on the sheet with the following titles:
   - location (or equipment type)
   - manufacturer
   - serial number
   - purchased or leased
   - first year of service
   - service contract
   - expiration date

4. Record the information for each piece of equipment, as available, in each row on the sheet.
   - Not all items will have a serial number. For this reason, some offices assign and attach an inventory number to each piece of equipment.
   - The lease or purchase date helps in identifying old equipment that may need to be replaced.
   - Service contracts should be tracked so managers can decide when and if to renew them.

5. Follow office policy in what you do with the completed inventory.

6. Update the inventory at regular intervals to show the following changes:
   - disposal of old equipment
   - addition of new equipment
   - relocation of equipment
   - renewal or expiration of service contracts

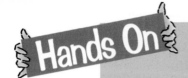

INVENTORY OF OFFICE SUPPLIES

3-4

It's important to keep track of supplies so your office doesn't run out of critical items, keep too much stock on hand, or use outdated medical supplies. Your office software can help you with this task. Follow these steps to use the computer to inventory supplies.

1. Open the spreadsheet software on your computer and create a document called *Supply Inventory*. If you use the computer when doing inventories, it will make calculating the use rate of supplies easier and more accurate.

2. Type the title of the file—for example, *Medical Supplies Inventory*—in the appropriate cell of the spreadsheet. You may want to inventory medical supplies and office supplies separately.

3. Create a row for each type of supply and columns across the spreadsheet to show the following data for each month of the year:
   • the amount on hand for that month
   • the amount used since the last inventory
   • the amount that needs to be ordered

4. Create formulas in the appropriate cells to automatically calculate the amount used and the number to be reordered.

5. Count the number of each item in the supply stock and record the number in the correct place on the spreadsheet.
   • As you count, check for supplies with expiration dates that have passed. Properly dispose of any such items. You should not use outdated supplies.
   • Pull items with the oldest expiration dates to the front of each type of supply. This will help to ensure that these items will be used first.

6. When the counts are complete and recorded on the spreadsheet, save your work and print out the spreadsheet.

7. Use the printed spreadsheet to reorder supplies. The spreadsheet formulas will have calculated how many of each item has been used and how many more you need to order.

8. When the new supplies arrive, stock them behind the existing supplies. This allows the oldest supplies to be used first.

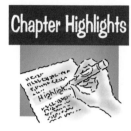

Chapter Highlights

- Computers are essential to the operation of a medical office.
- Computer software helps medical assistants do their jobs more efficiently.
- The Internet plays a key role in health care by providing medical information to patients and health care professionals.
- Quality improvement programs benefit medical offices by identifying potential problems and creating solutions for them.
- CLIA and HIPAA require attention to maintaining standards in both clinical and administrative areas of health care service.
- Risk management helps achieve quality improvement through the filing and review of incident reports.
- Medical assistants play key roles in maintaining equipment and supplies that are critical to a medical office.

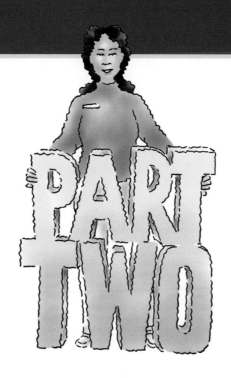

Administrative Skills

Chapter 4

MANAGING APPOINTMENTS AND SCHEDULES

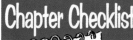

No medical office can run smoothly without a good system for scheduling appointments. This involves deciding when each patient will be seen and how much time to give her in the office. Do this well and you'll make good use of the physician's time and the office's resources. Do it poorly and confusion and chaos will rule. The result will be wasted time for patients, providers, and staff. You'll learn how to avoid these problems in this chapter.

Of course, every office will have emergencies, delays, and unexpected schedule changes. In this chapter, you'll also learn how to manage these challenges in an efficient and professional manner.

Appointment Scheduling Systems

There are two ways of scheduling appointments for patients.

- In a *manual system,* you'll write each patient's appointment into a book using a pencil or pen.
- In a *computerized system,* you'll use special software to schedule patients into an appointment book that is stored on your computer.

The method you use may depend on the size of the practice where you work. A large medical practice will have many providers who see patients by appointment. In some offices, these providers could include:

- physicians
- physicians' assistants
- nurse practitioners
- physical therapists
- other health care professionals

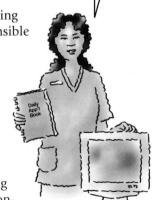

Whether you use a manual system or a computer for scheduling appointments, the guidelines are the same.

Some offices may have more than one person scheduling appointments. The number of providers you're responsible for may also determine which system you'll use.

MANUAL SCHEDULING

In some offices, you'll schedule appointments manually, even if the office's other systems are computerized.

The Appointment Book

To schedule patients in a manual system, the first thing you'll need is an appointment book. This book will contain enough pages to record all patient appointments over a set length of time—usually a year. You may want to see a week's appointments across the book's two facing pages when it's open. Or, you may prefer an appointment book with pages that show one day at a time.

Some appointment books even have a different color page for each day of the week. You would find this feature helpful if you had to flip forward in the book three weeks to make an appointment on a Wednesday, for instance.

If you work in an office with more than one provider, you'll probably be using an appointment book with a page for each day. Each page will have a column for each provider. If your office requires a lot of patient information when scheduling, your book's pages should be large enough to contain all the information.

In some offices, each doctor has his own appointment book. Appointment books come in many different colors and each physician can have a specific color.

APPOINTMENT BOOK STANDARDS

Any appointment book should meet these standards:

- It should be divided into units of time that are appropriate for your office. Some offices may schedule patients every 10 minutes. Other offices may prefer 15-minute or 20-minute intervals.
- The book should lie flat on your desk when you're using it. It should be easy to put back into its storage space when not in use.
- Each appointment space should be large enough for you to write in all the information your office requires. This should include *at least* the patient's name, phone number, and the reason for the visit.

The Matrix

Before scheduling appointments for a day, you'll need to set up a matrix for that day. You do this by crossing out the times providers are not available for appointments. Some of these times—such as lunch, for instance—may be the same every day. Other times providers are not available may repeat on the same day each week.

You'll have to block out other times, too, on a case-by-case basis, for vacations, business meetings, and so on. For instance, on the sample page, you can see that Dr. Smith has scheduled the afternoon off. It's also a good idea to block off time in each provider's schedule as "catch-up" time for emergencies and delays.

The appointment book is important for more than just scheduling appointments. Along with the notes in a patient's chart, it provides evidence of a patient's office visits. It also shows changes such as missed and rescheduled appointments. That information could help protect a physician in legal disputes like those you read about in Chapter 2.

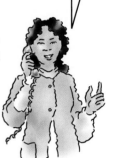

Leaving catch-up time in the schedule makes it easy for you to fit in last-minute appointments and emergency visits.

COMPUTERIZED SCHEDULING

Most software packages available for medical office management include a system for appointment scheduling. Using a computer to create schedules is helpful because it saves time. For example, you only have to enter routine information for a matrix one time—such as lunch everyday at noon, hospital rounds on Tuesdays from 9:00 A.M. to 11:00 A.M., and so on. You also can do these other things with just one click:

- add a patient
- add to the waiting list
- view a calendar
- search for available appointment times

To use the search feature, all you have to do is enter the date. The computer then shows the schedule for that day. Times available for appointments will be highlighted.

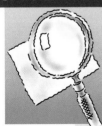

Closer Look   THE PATIENT APPOINTMENT BOOK

The reduced-size page at right shows patient appointments for one day in an office with three physicians.

- Notice that there is a column for each physician, plus a column for patients scheduled for blood tests in the lab.
- The matrix shows that Dr. Jones doesn't come in until 9:00 A.M. on Tuesdays. Dr. Stowe spends the morning seeing patients who are in the hospital. Dr. Jones goes to lunch at noon and the lab is closed for lunch between 1:00 P.M. and 2:00 P.M.

THURSDAY, APRIL 11

HOUR	Dr. Jones	Dr. Smith	Dr. Stowe	Lab
8:00	xxxxxxxxxxxxxxxxxxxx	Sue Dalton/555-2121 Recheck	xxx Hospital Rounds xxx	Jim Hunt/555-4332 FBS
8:15	xxxxxxxxxxxxxxxxxxxx	Dan Stevens/555-8515 Recheck	xxxxxxxxxxxxxxxxxxxx	Tony Bay/555-7899 FBS
8:30	xxxxxxxxxxxxxxxxxxxx	David Howell/555-7736	xxxxxxxxxxxxxxxxxxxx	Bob Taylor/555-6748
8:45	xxxxxxxxxxxxxxxxxxxx	back pain	xxxxxxxxxxxxxxxxxxxx	Shirley Teak/555-7746
9:00	Sam Johnson/555-2222	Jewel Cherry/555-4444	xxxxxxxxxxxxxxxxxxxx	Jenn Gibson/555-1137
9:15	CPE	CPE	xxxxxxxxxxxxxxxxxxxx	
9:30	I	I	xxxxxxxxxxxxxxxxxxxx	
9:45	?	?	xxxxxxxxxxxxxxxxxxxx	
10:00	Mandy Melton 555-1212/Recheck	Tony Disher/555-8812 Kindergarten PE	xxxxxxxxxxxxxxxxxxxx	
10:15	Diana Haris/555-4243 Recheck	I ?	xxxxxxxxxxxxxxxxxxxx	
10:30	Ray Ware/555-8321 suture removal	Joe South/555-3604 Recheck	xxxxxxxxxxxxxxxxxxxx	
10:45	Stan Gray/555-1708 Recheck		xxxxxxxxxxxxxxxxxxxx	
11:00	Jim Ashbaum/555-8512	xxxxxx catch up xxxxxx	xxxxxxxxxxxxxxxxxxxx	
11:15	suspicious rash	xxxxxxxxxxxxxxxxxxxx	xxxxxxxxxxxxxxxxxxxx	
11:30	xxxxxx catch up xxxxxx	Alice Cook 555-8561/Recheck	xxxxxxxxxxxxxxxxxxxx	
11:45	xxxxxxxxxxxxxxxxxxxx	Barry Stark/555-6731	xxxxxxxxxxxxxxxxxxxx	
12:00	xxxxxxx lunch xxxxxxx	high fever	xxxxxxxxxxxxxxxxxxxx	
12:15	xxxxxxxxxxxxxxxxxxxx		xxxxxxxxxxxxxxxxxxxx	
12:30	xxxxxxxxxxxxxxxxxxxx		xxxxxxxxxxxxxxxxxxxx	
12:45	xxxxxxxxxxxxxxxxxxxx	Sally Smart/555-3608 BP check	xxxxxxxxxxxxxxxxxxxx	
1:00		Bob Trasky/555-8754	Brad Melton/555-3284	xxxxxxx lunch xxxxxxx
1:15		stomach problems	Diabetes/New Pt.	xxxxxxxxxxxxxxxxxxxx
1:30			I	xxxxxxxxxxxxxxxxxxxx
1:45	Pat Silva/555-8888		?	xxxxxxxxxxxxxxxxxxxx
2:00	swollen glands	xxxxxxxx Off xxxxxxxx	Chas. Mallow/555-6739	
2:15	Jill Hill/555-9976	xxxxxxxxxxxxxxxxxxxx	immunizations	
2:30	Abscess (do not call)	xxxxxxxxxxxxxxxxxxxx		
2:45		xxxxxxxxxxxxxxxxxxxx		
3:00	Meet w/drug rep	xxxxxxxxxxxxxxxxxxxx		
3:15	about new antibiotic	xxxxxxxxxxxxxxxxxxxx	Bob Needles/555-1579	
3:30	I	xxxxxxxxxxxxxxxxxxxx	poss. sprained ankle	
3:45	I	xxxxxxxxxxxxxxxxxxxx		
4:00	?	xxxxxxxxxxxxxxxxxxxx		
4:15		xxxxxxxxxxxxxxxxxxxx		
4:30		xxxxxxxxxxxxxxxxxxxx		
4:45		xxxxxxxxxxxxxxxxxxxx		
5:00		xxxxxxxxxxxxxxxxxxxx	xxxxxx catch up xxxxxx	
5:15		xxxxxxxxxxxxxxxxxxxx	xxxxxxxxxxxxxxxxxxxx	
5:30		xxxxxxxxxxxxxxxxxxxx		
5:45		xxxxxxxxxxxxxxxxxxxx		
6:00	County Medical Society	xxxxxxxxxxxxxxxxxxxx	County Medical Society	
6:15	Meeting & Dinner	xxxxxxxxxxxxxxxxxxxx	Meeting & Dinner	
6:30	I	xxxxxxxxxxxxxxxxxxxx	I	
6:45	?	xxxxxxxxxxxxxxxxxxxx	?	
7:00				

NOTES

Another feature lets you search for the next available time slot. For example, suppose the physician tells a patient to return for a follow-up visit in two weeks. The patient wants an appointment after 1:00 P.M. Your computer will search for the first available time slot after 1:00 P.M., two weeks from that date. Some systems also let you search by the amount of time a visit is expected to take. So if a visit will require an hour, the computer will search only for those blocks of time that are 60 minutes or more.

The software also lets you print each day's schedule of appointments. In some offices, this schedule is known as the daily activity sheet. Other offices call it the day sheet.

Some scheduling software will also allow you to print billing slips and appointment reminders for patients. This gives you easy access to billing information. For example, when a patient calls for an appointment, you can remind him that he needs to pay his balance due of $32 when he comes for his next visit.

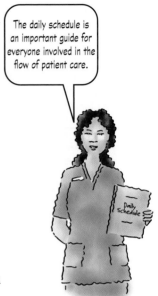

The daily schedule is an important guide for everyone involved in the flow of patient care.

Factors That Affect Scheduling

There's much more to scheduling appointments than just matching patients to time slots and hoping everything goes smoothly. Before you make an appointment, you should review the schedule and do the following:

- evaluate the patient's needs
- respect the physician's needs
- consider the office's limitations

THE PATIENTS' NEEDS

Most of the calls you will get to make appointments will be routine. But some patients may be shy or anxious. Others may be embarrassed or fearful about their medical problem. Be polite and professional as you collect the information you need. Here are some questions you should ask the patient when scheduling an appointment:

- Why do you wish to see the physician?
- Is the problem **acute** (a sudden onset) or **chronic** (longstanding)?

- How long have you had the symptoms?
- How severe are the symptoms?
- When is the best time for you to come in to the office? (Try to meet the patient's time requests, if you can. But don't overload the schedule.)
- Do you have any special needs, such as community van services, that we should keep in mind when making your appointment? (Some community van services operate only during certain hours.)
- Do you need to see other office staff while you're here?
- Does your insurance provider have any requirements that we should know about?

THE PROVIDERS' NEEDS

Managing appointments means more than just meeting patients' needs. To do your job well, you must meet the needs of the providers as well.

Some providers are very good about staying on schedule. Others often fall behind. This can cause backups in the reception area. Be aware of your providers' work patterns. To allow for her habits, your office manager or the provider may let you adjust how you schedule patients.

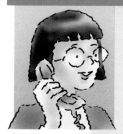

Ask the Professional   **MANAGING APPOINTMENTS**

Q: *A patient called the office last week and asked for an appointment next Monday at 1:00 P.M. Another patient was already scheduled then for a complete physical examination. But the caller said he could only come at 1:00, so I gave him the appointment anyway. Now the physician has to work this patient in. How could I have handled this situation better?*

A: It's your job to control the appointment schedule. You should have politely but firmly explained that 1:00 was already taken. You could have offered the patient another time on Monday or a 1:00 appointment on another day of the week. You also could have offered to put him on the "move-up" list if there is a cancellation for the time he wants. Remember, YOU control the schedule. Don't ever let it control you!

When you schedule appointments, you also must provide a physician time to:

- receive and return phone calls
- review lab reports and other test results
- dictate chart notes and letters
- meet with other physicians
- meet with sales people from drug companies and medical suppliers
- visit any patients he has admitted to the hospital

If the physician is on the staff of a teaching hospital, you may have to block off extra time for clinic conferences and other teaching duties.

Your job also may include clinical duties. You may have to remove sutures or give injections, for instance. That will affect the appointment schedule, too. Your clinical help probably will allow the physician to see more patients.

You should ask the physician how she wants to handle unscheduled office visitors who are not patients. For example, she may want to be told immediately if another physician comes to the office. She also may want another staff person to deal with sales people who drop by. Or she may ask you to schedule them for an appointment so she can talk with them at a more convenient time.

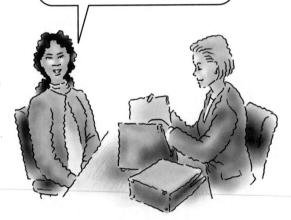

Salespeople will drop in frequently with information about new products and samples. Know your office's policy on handling sales calls.

PHYSICAL FACILITIES

The office's available facilities also will affect how you manage the appointment schedule. For example:

- How many providers are there?
- How many examination rooms are there?
- Is more than one set of instruments available, or must the same instruments be resterilized between procedures?
- How long does a procedure normally take?

You wouldn't schedule two sigmoidoscopies at the same time if there were only one room equipped for the procedure. Nor would you want to schedule the second patient 15 minutes later because the entire procedure may require 30 minutes.

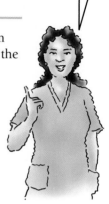

To help schedule appointments effectively, get to know all of the procedures the office staff performs.

Types of Scheduling

Most offices use some type of structured appointment system for scheduling visits. Patients are assigned a specific time on the schedule and allowed a set period for care. You'll probably use one of these methods for scheduling appointments:

- fixed scheduling
- streaming
- double booking
- wave and modified wave
- clustering

You also can combine some of these methods when making appointments.

FIXED SCHEDULING

You'll probably use some form of fixed scheduling. In fixed scheduling, each hour usually is divided into four 15-minute appointment slots. This is still the most common method of scheduling appointments. But if you don't do it well, fixed scheduling can have several disadvantages.

- *The patient may need more time than you scheduled.* You can help prevent this by finding out the patient's needs before you make the appointment. Knowing why the patient is coming to see the physician will tell you how many issues the physician must deal with. Then you can assign the number of time slots you think the patient will need. This practice is called **streaming**.

- *Patients who are late can disrupt the schedule by backing up the day's flow.* One way you can handle this is to schedule patients with a history of lateness toward the end of the day. You also can tell such patients to arrive 15 or 30 minutes before their actual scheduled time.

- *Patients who don't show up for their appointments can cause problems by wasting providers' time.* You can use **double booking** to avoid this problem.

Closer Look   HOW MUCH TIME TO ALLOW

A number of things can influence how much time you should allow for a patient's appointment. The office's size determines the number of examination rooms. The number of providers in the office is also a factor. Here are a few typical services and about how much time you should give for each.

- complete physical examination: one hour
- school physical: 30 minutes
- recheck: 15 minutes
- dressing change: 10 minutes
- blood pressure check: five minutes
- patient teaching: 30 minutes to one hour

Streaming

Streaming patients helps reduce schedule backups as well as gaps in time. You assign appointment lengths based on patients' needs. For example, you might give a patient coming in for a complete physical an hour-long appointment—that is, four 15-minute time slots. A patient in for a blood pressure check would get just one time slot, or 15 minutes. And you might even double book that time slot.

Double Booking

When you double book, you schedule two patients in the same time slot with the same physician. One sees the physician while the other goes for tests or is served by another applied health professional. Then they switch. When you use this method, the appointment slot isn't completely empty if one of the patients doesn't show up.

WAVE SCHEDULING

Many offices use a form of **wave scheduling** or change it in some way to fit their special needs. With wave scheduling, you schedule several patients for the same time. For example, you would give all patients to be seen in an hour the same appointment time, for instance, 11:00 A.M. Then, the physician takes the hour seeing these patients in the order they arrived.

The advantage of this system is that the physician isn't hurried to see patients at specific times. The disadvantage is that some patients may have long waits.

Modified Wave

The wave method has been modified, or changed, in many ways. One change is to fill the first half of each hour with one major appointment, such as a physical examination. In the second half hour, you would schedule three or four brief recheck or follow-up visits.

Here's another way you can use modified wave scheduling.

- Schedule half the number of patients the physician can see in an hour for the beginning of the hour.
- Schedule a third of the number of patients the physician can see in an hour at 20 minutes past the hour.
- Schedule the rest of the hour's patients at 40 minutes past the hour.

CLUSTERING

Clustering is the practice of grouping patients with similar problems or needs. Some medical offices reserve certain times or days for certain activities, such as physical examinations or other activities. For example, a pediatrician's office might have you schedule vaccinations only on certain days of the week. If you're working in an OB-GYN practice, the physicians might see pregnant patients in the mornings and other patients in the afternoons.

A

1:00	Larry Jones 555-4321 headaches
1:15	
1:30	Frank Ness 555-1234 follow up Rick Smith 555-8976 cast removal Nancy Wilson 555-7681 recheck throat Peter Paulson 555-9919 BP check
1:45	

B

1:00	Frank Ness 555-1234 follow up Dorothy Close 555-4321 CPE Larry Jones 555-3124 headaches
1:20	Rick Smith 555-8976 cast removal Nancy Wilson 555-7861 recheck throat
1:40	Peter Paulson 555-9919 BP check

These appointment schedules show two methods of modified wave scheduling. Note that one patient seen in method B could not be scheduled using method A. That's because a complete physical examination (CPE) is a major appointment, and method A allows only one major appointment per hour.

Secrets for Success   REMEMBERING APPOINTMENT TYPES

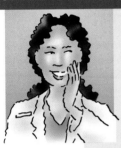

You can use the name of each type of appointment to help remember how it works.

- **Fixed Scheduling** Something that is "fixed" is stuck or attached to one place. In this method, patients are attached or stuck into one appointment slot.
- **Double Booking** Double means two. In this case, two patients are given the same appointment slot.
- **Streaming** Like rivers, some streams are long and others are short. When patients are streamed, their appointment times are of different lengths too.
- **Wave** Picture all patients arriving at once, as if they were being swept into the office on a big ocean wave.
- **Clustering** A "cluster" is things of the same kind that are bunched together. In clustering, patients with similar needs are seen in the same time period—bunched together in a "cluster."

Another use of clustering is that you might schedule certain tests, such as sigmoidoscopies, only at certain times of the week. Clustering has several advantages.

- It makes the best use of special equipment.
- Patients with similar problems can be educated at the same time.
- The schedule is easier to manage.
- It makes the use of staff time more efficient.

You can combine clustering with fixed scheduling, wave scheduling, or modified wave. You also can combine double booking with this and other forms of scheduling.

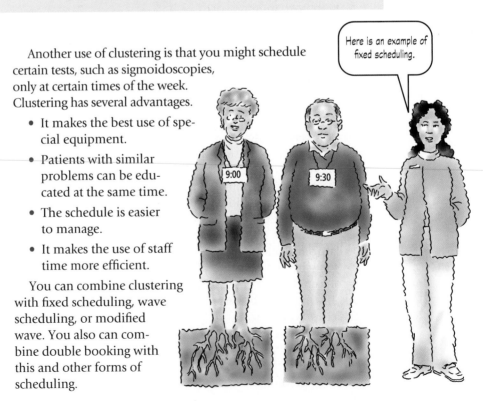

Here is an example of fixed scheduling.

Scheduling Guidelines

Some patients will call for appointments. Others will schedule their appointments in person. Whatever the method, you always should be professional, pleasant, and helpful.

Leave a few open appointment times in the morning and again in the afternoon. Late arrivals and other delays often will upset the schedule. These open time slots can help the schedule "catch up" again. They also create time for emergencies, last-minute appointments, or walk-in patients.

APPOINTMENTS FOR NEW PATIENTS

Most appointments for new patients are made by telephone. You must have very good communication with the patient at this time. It's critical that you record the patient's information accurately.

It is likely that your office will have its own procedures for making new patient appointments. Some offices might even have you follow a script to make sure it's done right. The Hands On feature on page 160 gives you some general guidelines.

If there's enough time before the appointment, mail an office brochure to the patient. Some offices send a new-patient form as well. The patient can complete it and bring it in at the appointment. It saves time if the form doesn't have to be filled out at the office.

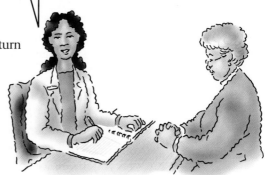

Always write the patient's phone number on the appointment schedule. Emergencies happen, and schedule changes are easier if the patient's phone number is handy.

APPOINTMENTS FOR ESTABLISHED PATIENTS

The physician may tell a patient to return for a follow-up visit. Most return appointments are made before the patient leaves the office. The Hands On feature on page 161 outlines the steps to follow in making a return appointment.

The Daily Schedule

In most offices, you'll be asked to prepare a daily schedule of appointments. You can use computer scheduling software to print out these schedules.

Make a schedule for each provider with copies for other staff members. Place the next day's schedule on the physician's desk before she leaves for the day. Give next week's schedule to the physician before she leaves on Friday.

You should include the following information on these schedules:

- the next day's patient appointments
- the physician's hospital rounds
- the physician's surgery schedule
- any professional or business meetings
- any personal appointments that are on the schedule

If you work in an office that uses computer scheduling, you may need to create and print a weekly schedule as well. Many offices create a weekly schedule in case of a computer "crash" that erases important information. If you have a weekly schedule printed, you will still have a fairly accurate record of appointments.

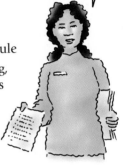

The schedule may change as the day progresses. Remember to give everyone any corrected copies of the schedule that you distribute.

Patient Reminders

Patients are less likely to miss an appointment when they are reminded of it. Medical offices use appointment cards, telephone calls, e-mails, and mailed cards to help patients remember upcoming visits.

APPOINTMENT CARDS

You should give the patient a card showing his next appointment when he leaves the office. The card should have the following information on it:

- the patient's name
- the day, date, and time of the next visit
- the physician's name and phone number

Computer scheduling software also can print appointment cards for you. If you write them by hand, use ink that can't be erased.

If the patient needs a series of appointments, try to make them for the same time and on the same day of the week. If there's space on the card, you could list the whole series of appointments on it. But it's probably better to give the patient a card for his next visit only. Just give him a new card after each visit.

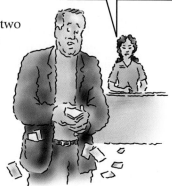

Only give a patient one appointment card at a time. Handing out all the cards for a series of visits can lead to confusion and lost cards.

TELEPHONE REMINDERS

Patients also should get a telephone reminder or confirmation call one or two days before their appointment. Some computer scheduling software will call patients automatically with a recorded reminder message.

Whether you make the call or whether it's made by computer, call only the patient's home number. Don't call a work number unless the patient asks you to do so. Document the patient's preferences in the chart so everyone in the office can see this information.

Federal privacy laws allow you to leave an appointment reminder message on a patient's answering machine or with whoever answers their home phone. But it's still a good idea to ask the patient if that is okay. You should ask at the time you make the appointment.

Don't leave a message on a patient's work phone or with a coworker, even if the patient has asked you to call her there. Leaving a message at work isn't a good idea. It raises privacy concerns that usually don't exist when you make reminder calls to the patient's home.

Don't ever include the reason for the visit in a reminder message. If a person answers the phone and wants more information, politely decline to give it. Tell the person that patient privacy issues don't allow you to answer the question.

SAMPLE TELEPHONE REMINDER

Your reminder call should be brief. Simply state your name, your office, and the date and time of the appointment. For example, you might say:

- "This is Ms. Palmer from Dr. Reid's office. I'm calling to confirm your appointment for tomorrow, Thursday, February 10, at 3:30 P.M."

- Unless the patient has a question, just say, "Thank you and goodbye."

(continued)

- You should write "confirmed," "left message," or "no answer" on the appointment schedule to show the results of each call.

Recorded messages left by the computer should have the same basic content. They should include a call-back number if the patient can't keep the appointment. Include a call-back number when you leave a reminder message, too.

REMINDER CARDS

Your office may send reminder cards or letters instead of making phone calls. These cards also can be used for patients who don't want phone reminders. You should mail the reminder card at least a week before the appointment date.

Some offices use reminder cards to alert patients that it's time for some annual exam, such as a Pap smear, mammogram, prostate exam, or complete physical. For privacy reasons, however, the reminder card should never state the kind of exam. It should have a general message printed on it. Here's an example:

"According to our records, you are due for your annual visit. Please call the office and we will be glad to make an appointment for you."

For privacy reasons, some patients may want their reminder cards mailed inside an envelope. This is a reasonable request, and you should go along with it. You also should accommodate a patient who wants the card mailed to some place other than his home.

Reminder calls and cards help patients remember their appointments. If they need to cancel or reschedule, you may be able to fill that slot with another patient. Keep a list of names and phone numbers of patients who have asked to be called if an earlier appointment becomes available. You might call this a cancellation list, a waiting list, or a move-up list in your office.

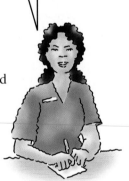

Write only the appointment date and time on the reminder card, never the reason for the visit. Remember, you have no way of knowing who will see the card after it's been mailed.

Laila Hudson

has an appointment with

DONALD L. MYERS, M.D.
NEUROLOGICAL SURGERY
233 SOUTH SIXTH STREET, FIRST FLOOR
PHILADELPHIA, PENNSYLVANIA 19106
(215) 627-4380
on

<u>2:00</u> , <u>Tues.</u> , <u>April</u>   <u>8</u> , 200 <u>7</u>
time   weekday   month   date

If your plans change please notify the office at least 24 hours in advance

Adapting the Schedule

It will be an unusual day in the office if everything goes according to plan. Often, patients will be late for appointments or even miss them altogether. Providers may experience delays. Patients who don't have appointments may call the office with emergencies. You may have to adjust the appointment schedule when these things happen.

EMERGENCIES

When a patient calls with an emergency, first find out whether the problem can be treated in the office. Every office should have a policy for evaluating emergency calls.

Headed for the ER

Follow your office policy. But in general, you should put through to the office nurse or physician any caller who complains of these symptoms:

- chest pain
- shortness of breath
- loss of consciousness
- severe bleeding
- severe vomiting or diarrhea
- temperature greater than 102 degrees

Most likely, patients with these symptoms need to be seen in a hospital emergency room (ER).

Seen in the Office

Here are some typical symptoms that would require the patient to be seen in the office the same day. Again, the policy in your office will be the final word on how to handle these cases.

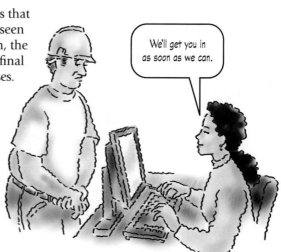

- severe vomiting for more than two days
- high fever for more than two days
- severe headache with neck stiffness
- abdominal pain with symptoms of appendicitis
- wounds that don't require a trip to the ER

Closer Look   CONSTELLATION OF SYMPTOMS

When certain symptoms happen together, it can signal a specific problem. Such a group of complaints is called a **constellation of symptoms.** Keep the following in mind:

- Severe pain in the lower right abdomen, nausea, and fever is the constellation of symptoms for appendicitis.
- Chest pain, shortness of breath, arm or neck pain, and nausea and/or vomiting is the constellation of symptoms for a heart attack.
- Severe headache, dizziness, trouble speaking or seeing, and numbness or weakness of the face, arm, or leg is the constellation of symptoms for a stroke.

If a patient needs to be seen the same day and no appointments are available, you can adapt the schedule in three possible ways:

- Work in the patient between existing appointments. This will result in delays for patients with appointments that follow, but the emergency may need to be addressed immediately.
- Put the patient in an open slot you have created as catch-up time in the schedule. Keep in mind that some emergencies may require quicker attention, however.
- Schedule the patient into a filled time slot, then call that person and reschedule his appointment. Explain that an emergency requires you to do this. This may not be a good alternative, however, if the emergency patient needs to be seen quickly.

ACUTELY ILL PATIENTS

You'll also receive calls from patients who are seriously ill but don't have a true emergency. These patients need to be seen as soon as possible, but not necessarily that very day. You should triage these calls in this way:

- Get as much information about the patient's problem as you can. Write a note containing this information. This will help the physician decide when the patient should be seen.

- Place the patient's chart with the note in the place the physician has chosen for such calls.
- Tell the patient you'll call back as soon as the physician makes a decision.

Once again, your office policy will determine how calls like this are handled. Here are some examples of complaints from patients who need to be seen soon, although not necessarily that very day.

- severe sore throat
- severe back pain
- burning and/or painful urination
- headache lasting more than three days
- jaundice that has appeared in the last week
- severe respiratory symptoms of more than a week
- severe rash lasting more than three days
- heart palpitations for more than two days

IT'S THE PHYSICIAN'S CALL

If the physician wants to see the patient, he will tell you how soon. You can adjust the schedule using the same system you use to work in emergency patients.

Acutely ill patients don't need to be seen as quickly, however. So if you must cancel a scheduled appointment to work in an acutely ill patient, try not to do it for the same day. This is because you might not be able to reach the patient you're canceling in time. You do not want that person showing up in the office only to find that her appointment was cancelled. But if you cancel an appointment for the next day, you can call the patient's home and leave a message that she'll probably get.

Most importantly, remember that the physician or the triage nurse always should make the final decision when adjusting the schedule for an emergency.

OTHER SCHEDULE BUSTERS

Other events that will require you to adapt the schedule may be more common.

Just Walk On In

Walk-ins are patients who come to the office without an appointment. Your office may have a procedure for handling these patients. But in general, you must first find out why the patient has come in. If it's an emergency, the patient should be seen immediately. Otherwise, have the patient sit in the waiting room while you tell the physician. The physician can then decide whether to see the patient or ask him to make an appointment.

If the physician is going to see the patient, explain that you'll work him in as soon as possible. When the patient leaves after being seen, apologize for the delay. Suggest that he make an appointment next time.

I'm Late! I'm Late! For a Very Important Date!

Patients who are late can cause problems in the schedule for the rest of the day. You should remind the patient gently but firmly that she was late and tell her the physician is with another patient. Offer the patient the choice of waiting or rescheduling the appointment.

Some offices have a policy requiring that patients who are more than 15 minutes late be rescheduled. Of course, late patients may not always be a problem. If the physician is running behind, a late patient may have arrived before it's his turn to be seen.

One thing you might do is schedule patients who have a habit of being late toward the end of the day. That way, their lateness will affect the day's schedule less. Also, you can ask patients to call the office if they know they are going to be late.

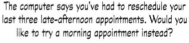

The computer says you've had to reschedule your last three late-afternoon appointments. Would you like to try a morning appointment instead?

Always call patients with a history of being late to remind them of their appointment. You should do this even if it's not normally office policy to make appointment reminders by phone.

The Trouble with No-Shows

A no-show occurs when a patient misses an appointment and doesn't call the office ahead of time. When this happens, try to call the patient to find out why the appointment was missed. Then, try to reschedule the patient for another day.

Legal Brief   DOCUMENTING NO-SHOWS

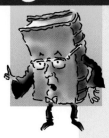

It's essential that information about no-shows be documented in the chart as well as on the daily schedule. Use red ink when marking a no-show on the daily schedule and the patient's chart.

You should make notes in the patient's record of all actions involving missed appointments. Copies of any letters sent to the patient should be included in the chart too.

The information in both the appointment schedule and patient's chart must look the same. This is vital information for legal issues as well as for the patient's welfare.

If you cannot reach the patient by phone, send a card asking him to call the office to reschedule. Write in the patient's chart that the appointment was missed. Also, note if you rescheduled the appointment or mailed a card for the patient to reschedule.

Tell the physician about patients who continually miss appointments. She may want to call the patient or send a letter of concern for the patient's welfare. This is especially true for patients who are seriously ill. In extreme cases, the physician may want to end her relationship with the patient. The procedure for doing this is discussed in Chapter 2.

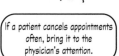

Call patients who've missed past appointments the day before their scheduled visit, just like you would call frequently late patients.

I'm Calling to Cancel

Here's what to do when a patient cancels an appointment.

- Ask the patient why she is canceling.
- Mark the cancellation on the appointment schedule.
- Note the cancellation and the reason in the patient's chart.
- Offer to reschedule the appointment at another time.

If the physician is seeing the patient for a continuing medical concern, make sure the patient understands the importance of rescheduling. The patient may say she'll call later to reschedule. Make a note to yourself to check on the call-back in a few days.

If a patient cancels and you have a full schedule, no action is needed. But if the schedule is light, use your move-up list to try to fill the opening.

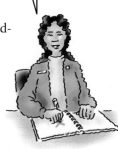

If a patient cancels appointments often, bring it to the physician's attention.

Closer Look   DOCUMENTING MISSED APPOINTMENTS

You should note missed appointments, whether they're cancellations or no-shows, in the patient's chart. Also, include a summary of the reason for the missed appointment. Below is a sample of one such note in a patient's chart:

Mrs. Parrish was called regarding missing scheduled appointment for today at 9:30 A.M. Patient said she forgot about the appointment. Appointment was rescheduled for 10/15/07 at 10:00 A.M. Patient was advised of the need to have regular prenatal checkups. Patient verbalized understanding. Dr. Wong was notified that appointment was missed and rescheduled.–Noreen Brooks, CMA

OFFICE CANCELLATIONS

The office may have to cancel patients' appointments if the doctor is ill, has an emergency, or takes personal time off. Patients don't need to be told the specific reason for the physician's absence. Cancellation by the office should be noted in a patient's record too. Here are some guidelines to follow:

- *If you have advance notice:* Write a letter to patients with appointments you must cancel. Simply state that the physician will be away from the office and will return by a certain date. Ask the patient to call the office to reschedule. Remember to place a copy of the letter in the patient's chart.

- *If you must cancel on the day of the appointment:* Call the patient. Explain that the physician has been called out of the office unexpectedly. Try to reschedule the appointment while the patient is still on the phone.

- *If the patient arrives before you can contact him:* Apologize and politely explain the situation. Most patients will be understanding.

When the physician won't be available for a long time, another physician must cover the practice or be on call. If a substitute physician is employed, office appointments won't be disrupted.

You also should have a list of the names and addresses of physicians who are on call to see patients. Give this information to patients you must cancel, if your office policy allows it.

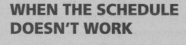

Running Smoothly

WHEN THE SCHEDULE DOESN'T WORK

You've been doing everything right. You follow office procedures for scheduling new and established patients. You remind patients of their appointments. You're using scheduling strategies with frequently late patients, and you try hard to fill slots created by cancellations. You expect that some days will not run smoothly. But the schedule seems in chaos almost every day, and you just can't figure out why.

This situation is a case where a study might help. Here's what to do:

- Look at the schedule over the past two or three months.
- List all the patients seen, when they arrived, how long they spent with the physician, and when they left the office.

Your study might show that many patients are arriving late, or that not enough time is being allowed for certain procedures. Perhaps too many staff members are allowed to make patient appointments. Maybe a frequently late physician is part of the problem.

Some problems may never be solved completely. But if you can identify them, you often can make changes so their effects will be less severe.

The Doctor Has Been Delayed

Sometimes the physician will arrive late to the office. If his appointment hours have not yet started, call patients with early appointments. Give them the choice of coming in later or on another day.

If patients are waiting, tell them at once that the physician has been delayed. Also tell them how long the delay is expected to be. Ask if they want to wait or reschedule for another time. If patients reschedule, be sure to note the reason in their chart.

> Always keep patients informed about delays. Most will understand if they know you haven't forgotten them.

Appointments with Other Providers

The physician may want a patient to see another doctor, perhaps a specialist in another field of medicine. The patient also may need to be sent to another office or facility for testing or to be admitted to the hospital. In each case, you may need to make the appointment with the other provider.

Two's a Party—Three's a Crowd!

In making an outside appointment, you must first be sure it meets the requirements of **third-party payers.** These are the insurance companies, HMOs, and other health care plans that pay patients' medical bills.

You'll read more about third-party payers in Chapter 8 when you learn about processing health insurance. For now, you should know that managed-care companies, such as HMOs, have guidelines for sending patients to other providers. The requirements are called **precertification.** This means the insurer must approve the appointment in advance.

Call the phone number on the patient's insurance card before making these kinds of appointments:

- sending the patient to another physician
- scheduling certain tests or procedures
- admitting the patient to the hospital (This only applies to admissions that are *not* emergencies.)

My Provider Is Preferred

Be sure the provider you're calling is a **preferred provider** for the patient's health care plan. These are physicians, hospitals, and others that are in the plan's approved network of providers.

Unless you send the patient to a preferred provider, the plan's payment will be less. Also, if a referral, test, or hospitalization requires precertification and you don't have it, the health care plan may not pay at all. In each case, both the patient and your employer could suffer financial losses.

CONSULTATIONS AND REFERRALS

Sometimes the physician will want you to schedule a **consultation** or a **referral** for a patient. You need to know the difference between the two. In a consultation, the physician wants another physician's opinion about the patient. The second physician reviews the patient's records and usually examines the patient. He then recommends treatment.

- In a *consultation*, the patient's physician carries out the treatment, not the other physician. One required part of a

Closer Look   PRECERTIFICATION

A health care plan will want certain information before granting approval to send a patient to another provider. Each plan will be different. But in general, you should have this information ready when you call a patient's plan for approval:

- the information on the patient's plan ID card
- the patient's name, address, phone number, and age
- if the patient is a family member of the insured, her relationship to the insured
- the name, address, and phone number of the provider asking for the approval
- the name, address, and phone number of the provider to whom the patient will be sent
- the patient's diagnosis or symptoms
- the type of care being sought
- if the patient is being admitted to a hospital, the name, address, and phone number of the hospital

You will need to get the health care plan's approval first, unless the patient is being sent as an emergency case. In that case, you should call for approval as soon as you can.

consultation is a consultation letter or report from the consultant to the primary care physician.

- In a *referral*, the patient's care and treatment is actually transferred to the other physician.

The Hands On procedure on page 162 shows the steps to follow when making appointments for consultations and referrals. In some cases, the patient will want to make his own appointment with the other physician. If so, ask the patient to call you when the appointment is made. Write the date and time the patient gives you in the patient's chart.

DIAGNOSTIC TESTS

A physician in your office may want to send a patient to another facility for testing. The steps in the Hands On procedure on page 162 apply to making these appointments too. You'll make some of these appointments while the patient is still in the office. This is especially true for labs tests and x-rays. Check with the patient for any scheduling conflicts she might have.

Some tests, such as CT scans and MRIs, may require precertification by the patient's health plan.

Testing, Testing!

Some of the tests you might send a patient out for are:

- laboratory tests (mainly blood tests)
- radiology (x-rays)
- computed tomography (CT scans)
- magnetic resonance imaging (MRIs)
- nuclear medicine studies

Getting Results!

Find out exactly what test or tests the physician wants and how soon she needs the results. Give the patient a lab or x-ray referral slip with the requested tests marked on it. Be sure to tell the provider if the results are needed STAT, or immediately. Also give the patient a slip with the outside facility's name, address, and phone number, and the date and time of his appointment.

Some tests may require advance preparation by the patient. Tell him what he must do, and also give him written instructions. Be sure he understands the importance of following them.

Write the appointment time and date and the name of the outside facility on the patient's chart. Also, put a reminder note in your appointment schedule to check for when the test results are back.

SCHEDULING SURGERIES

You also may have to schedule procedures in a hospital operating room or an outpatient surgery center. You may have to get precertification for these from the patient's health care plan too. Follow the same general steps in the Hands On procedure on page 162 that you do for referrals and testing.

When scheduling surgeries, you'll need to follow these additional steps as well.

- Tell the surgical facility the exact procedure, the type of anesthesia required, and the time needed. The physician will provide this information. Also, give the facility any other information and instructions your physician provides.
- Provide the patient's age, health care plan, and the plan's approval number for the surgery.

- Give patients going to a hospital a preadmission form, if you have a supply from the hospital in your office.
- Be sure to follow the policies of the hospital or outpatient facility about preadmission testing. These may include blood tests, x-rays, and a donation of the patient's own blood in advance.
- List all the appointment dates, times, and places the patient needs to go. Give this list to the patient. Make sure the patient understands where to go, when, and what will happen in each place.
- Finally, write the name of the surgical facility and the date and time the surgery is scheduled in the patient's chart. You may need to arrange for hospital admission by providing this information to the hospital admitting department.

The Physician's Schedule

Your scheduling duties will extend to the physicians in the office as well as the patients. You probably will help manage the physician's professional schedule. This includes allowing time in the appointment schedule for the physician's other professional activities. It also may involve making travel arrangements for the physician.

MANAGING THE PHYSICIAN'S TIME

You already are helping manage the physician's time when you create the matrix for the appointment schedule. The matrix sets time aside for the physician's activities outside the office, including surgeries and hospital rounds.

Another duty may be to screen visitors, including salespeople, for the physician.

- *Pharmaceutical sales representatives.* These visitors can be a valuable resource for a physician. They provide information about new drugs that are available. Ask the physician for a list of pharmaceutical sales reps he wants to see. This probably will depend on the physician's specialty. A cardiologist and a psychiatrist would not be interested in the same kinds of drugs, for instance.
- *Medical suppliers.* These people are another valuable source of information. But which suppliers are worth seeing also depends on the physician's specialty. For example, an

internal medicine doctor wouldn't want to spend time with a supplier of artificial hips and knees.

- *Office suppliers and suppliers of medical forms.* The office manager usually handles these types of visitors. They should not be allowed to take up the physician's time unless she wants to see them. The same is true of insurance salespeople.

- *Community leaders and fundraisers.* These visitors may arrive to ask for the physician's support for some local project. Your medical office probably has a general policy for handling them. Find out if the physician wishes to be notified of these types of visitors. Bluntly refusing to help is not good for community relations. Instead, you might tell them of the physician's current community activities. If appropriate, explain that he cannot take on any more at this time.

MAKING TRAVEL ARRANGEMENTS

Many physicians attend professional meetings and educational conferences to keep current in their field. You may have to make arrangements for physicians in your office to attend such events.

Create a one-page travel profile for each physician. Here's the information you'll need:

- the names and phone numbers of travel agents the physician likes to use

- the airline(s) on which the physician likes to travel. Include his frequent flier number(s), preferred class (for example, first class or coach), seating preference (for example, aisle or window seat), and ticket preference (paper ticket or ticketless travel).

- rental car preferences, including the rental company and type of car preferred (compact, standard, SUV, luxury, etc.)

- preferred hotel accommodations, including price range, bed size, and features (swimming pool, restaurant, fitness facility, etc.)

- the physician's or office's credit card number(s)

When the physician tells you that she wishes to attend a certain conference, complete the registration form as soon as possible. Once you have confirmed the physician is registered, make the travel arrangements. You may do this through a travel agent. Or you might make the reservations yourself using the Internet. In either case, use the information from the physician's travel profile to arrange a flight, hotel, and, if needed, a rental car.

If you use a travel agent, he will provide an **itinerary.** This is a detailed plan of the trip. You will need at least three copies of the itinerary.

- Give the first copy to the physician to carry on the trip.
- The second copy is for the physician to leave with his family.
- Keep the third copy in the office, in case you need to contact the physician.

BEING YOUR OWN ONLINE TRAVEL AGENT

If you make the travel arrangements using the Internet, you will have to prepare the itinerary yourself. Here's what you should include:

- *Air travel:* the date of the flight, airport, airline, flight and seat number, and departure and arrival times. Unless the flight is nonstop, do the same for the connecting flight(s). You also will need to provide this information for the return trip.
- *Rental car:* the rental company's name and phone number, reservation confirmation number, and type of car reserved
- *Hotel:* the name and address, phone number, reservation confirmation number, and dates of the stay
- *Meeting or conference:* name, location address and phone number, room number, and registration confirmation number

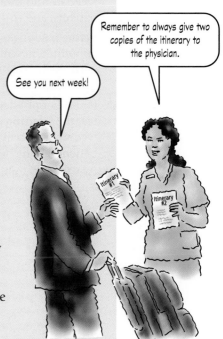

Be sure to get confirmation numbers when making hotel and rental car reservations. If the physician is flying with a paper ticket, check it when it arrives. The dates, flight numbers, and times should match those on the itinerary you prepared.

Put two copies of the itinerary, a copy of the conference registration form, and the ticket (or airline e-mail for ticketless travel) into an envelope and give it to the physician. Then, all that's left is to wish her a good trip!

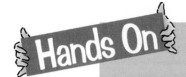

Follow these steps when making an appointment for a new patient.

1. Obtain the patient's full name, address, day and evening phone numbers, reason for the visit, and name of who referred the patient. This information helps you determine how soon and for how long the patient will need to be seen.

2. Explain the office's payment policy. Ask the patient to bring insurance information to the office. Patients cannot be expected to make any required payments unless they are aware of the policy.

3. Make sure the patient knows where the office is located. Give directions if needed. This helps patients arrive on time.

4. Ask the patient if it's acceptable to call them at home or work. Some patients don't want medically related messages left on voicemail or with a coworker.

5. Double-check your appointment book or computer screen to make sure you have recorded the appointment for the correct date and time. Mistakes can cause overbooking, angry patients, and irritated physicians and staff.

6. Before hanging up, confirm the day, date, and time of the appointment with the patient. Repeating this information ensures that no mistakes or misunderstandings have occurred.

7. If another physician referred the patient, make a note to contact the referring physician's office for copies of the patient's records. This will give the physician information about the patient that he needs. It also may eliminate the need to repeat some tests.

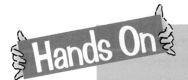

MAKING APPOINTMENTS FOR ESTABLISHED PATIENTS

4-2

Follow these steps to schedule a return appointment.

1. Find out the reason for the return visit. If a specific test is to be done, check the schedule to see when the equipment is available. This will help you offer a good date and time.

2. Offer the patient a specific date and time. If the patient doesn't agree, offer one or two other dates and times. Just asking the patient, "When would you like to return?" can create indecision in the patient.

3. Enter the patient's name and telephone contact number in the appointment book or the computer. Having this information with the appointment makes it easier to call the patient if you have to cancel or reschedule it.

4. Place the information on an appointment card and give it to the patient. Repeat aloud to the patient the day, date, and time of the appointment as you hand over the card. This step helps the patient remember the appointment.

5. Double-check your record of the appointment to be sure you have not made an error. Appointment errors waste time for everyone, including the patient, staff, and physician.

6. End your conversation with a pleasant word and smile. Your friendliness will feel good to a patient who may be anxious about having to return to the physician.

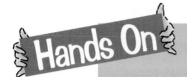

MAKING APPOINTMENTS FOR PATIENTS IN OTHER FACILITIES

4-3

The steps for arranging referrals, testing and other procedures, or hospitalization are much the same. Follow these guidelines when making arrangements.

1. Make certain that the requirements of the patient's health care plan are met. Many health plans require that referrals to specialists, hospital admissions, certain diagnostic tests, and surgical procedures be approved in advance. The phone numbers to call will be printed on the patient's insurance card.

2. Refer to the preferred provider list for the patient's health care plan and call a provider on this list. Many plans have lists of approved physicians, hospitals, and other facilities that patients must use. If there's more than one approved provider, let the patient choose from the list if she wishes.

3. Have the following information available when you call the provider:
   - the name and phone number of your office and physician
   - the patient's name, address, and phone number
   - the reason the patient is being sent to the other provider
   - how urgent it is that the patient be seen
   - the approval number from the patient's health care plan if precertification is required

   This information allows the other provider to serve the patient's needs.

4. Record the following information in the patient's chart when you make the call:
   - the date and time of the call
   - the name of the person you spoke with

   You need this record to document the patient's care.

5. Ask the person you're calling to notify you if the patient doesn't keep the appointment. If this happens, tell the physician and record the missed appointment in the patient's chart. This information also helps document the patient's care.

6. Write the following on office stationery and give or mail it to the patient:
   - the name, address, and phone number of the place you are sending the patient
   - the date and time of the patient's appointment at this place

   This gives the patient a reminder so the appointment will be kept.

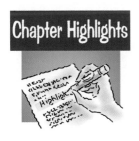

Chapter Highlights

- A medical office needs a good and well-managed appointment system to run smoothly and efficiently.
- Scheduling systems include manual ones that use appointment books and computerized ones that use special software.
- Computerized systems make it easier to meet the scheduling needs of patients and providers and to produce updated daily schedules.
- The number of providers, a facility's size, and the services it offers all influence the scheduling system and methods that work best.
- Methods used to schedule appointments include fixed, double booking, streaming, clustering, wave, and modified wave.
- Scheduling appointments for new and returning patients requires meeting both the patient's and the provider's needs.
- Appointment cards, phone reminders, and reminder cards make patients less likely to miss their appointments.
- On many days, emergencies, delays, late patients, walk-ins, cancellations, and no-shows will require schedule adjustments.
- Some health care plans may place special requirements on sending the patients they cover to other providers.
- Extra steps may be needed when scheduling patients for certain tests, surgical procedures, or hospital admissions.
- In addition to scheduling appointments, you also may help with organizing the physician's schedule and travel plans.

Chapter 5

DOCUMENTATION

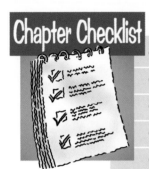

Chapter Checklist

- List the kinds of information contained in a medical record

- Establish and maintain the medical record

- Contrast the ways in which medical records can be organized

- Organize a patient's medical record

- Explain how to make entries in a patient's medical record

- Describe how to make corrections in medical records

- Document appropriately

- Describe the ways medical records can be filed and stored

- File medical records

- Compare standard and electronic medical record systems

Working with patients' medical records is one of the most important jobs you'll have as a medical assistant. A fair amount of your time will be spent writing in, adding items to, filing, or retrieving patients' charts. A medical record is a form of communication as well as a legal document. It provides information about a patient's health to those who read it while providing evidence of the care the patient has received.

Good medical records are vital to the smooth operation of any medical office. Physicians and other staff must be able to locate a patient's chart quickly, as well as the desired information inside it. In this chapter, you'll learn how to organize and maintain patient records. You'll also learn about managing medical records systems.

On the Record

Medical records are a critical part of health care. In some settings, a patient's medical record may be referred to as a *chart* or a *file*. But no matter what it's called, it's the history of a patient's involvement with your office. It's the official record of the following things:

- the physician's evaluation of the patient's health
- treatments carried out on the patient
- changes in the patient's medical condition
- communication between the patient and the staff

Medical records have other uses, too. For example, they can be valuable for research, in creating quality improvement (QI) programs, and for patient education. Information from medical records also helps the government protect the public's health as well as plan for future health care needs.

MEDICAL RECORDS AND YOU

You will deal with medical records nearly every day—writing in them, adding lab reports and other items, and so on. Patients' charts must meet certain legal and ethical standards. So must your work with them. Unorganized medical records can expose the office to embarrassment and possibly even lawsuits. Much of the responsibility for preventing these types of problems will be in your hands.

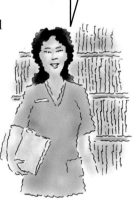

Taking good care of patients' charts can help protect your office against lawsuits.

The standard way of keeping medical records is to have a paper folder for each patient. The reports, forms, and other information resulting from the patient's office visits are organized inside this folder.

In recent years, some offices have begun keeping patients' charts on the computer. But no matter how your office stores patients' medical records, the information in them must be:

- easy to retrieve
- kept in an orderly manner
- accurate and complete
- brief

Your skills in organizing and maintaining patients' charts will play a big part in whether the records meet these standards.

PATIENT CHARTS 101

Here are two basic things you need to know about chart organization.

1. A medical record contains two types of information.

   - *Personal information.* This includes the patient's name, address, telephone number, date of birth, social security number, and next of kin. Many offices also include a photocopy of the patient's health insurance card.

   - *Clinical information.* This is the information about the patient's health, medical conditions, and treatment.

2. Never mix the patient's clinical information with his or her personal information.

   - In a paper chart, clinical information is fastened to one side of the open folder.

   - The personal information is attached to the other side.

CLINICAL COMPONENTS OF THE PATIENT'S CHART

Here's the kind of information you usually will find in the clinical part of a patient's chart. The first five items form what is called the History and Physical (H&P) part of the chart. They're generally recorded on a preprinted form called the progress notes.

- *chief complaint*—the patient's explanation of why he came to see the doctor, usually stated in the patient's own words, in quotation marks

- *present illness*—the patient's complaint stated in medical terms, with times and details

- *medical history*—a review of major illnesses of parents and grandparents, aunts and uncles, and brothers and sisters, as well as the patient's major illnesses and surgeries. This section is sometimes called *family and personal history.*

- *review of systems*—an examination of the patient's ten major body systems to look for problems not yet identified

- *diagnosis* or *medical impression*—the physician's opinion of the patient's medical problems

- *progress notes*—a record of what happened each time the patient was seen, including phone calls and prescription refills. The progress notes usually begin with the patient's H&P information.

- *radiographic reports*—reports of x-rays, CT scans, MRIs, and similar studies that were done in the office or at another facility

- *laboratory results*—copies of the results of any tests done at the office or at an outside facility. Examples might include blood work and electrocardiographs (EKGs).
- *consultation reports*—reports from other physicians with whom the patient's physician asked to consult about the patient
- *medication administration*—a record of the medicines the patient was given or prescribed. Some offices use a separate sheet for any injections and other medication the patient received in the office.
- *all correspondence*—copies of any letters or memos the office sent about the patient, copies of any letters from the patient, and correspondence from other physicians
- *miscellaneous*—consent forms and the HIPAA privacy notice signed by the patient, as well as copies of any patient instructions regarding end-of-life decisions. These might include organ donation forms, a living will, and a power of attorney for health care.

Closer Look   ELECTRONIC MEDICAL RECORDS

As you read in Chapter 3, computers play an important role in running a medical office. In recent years, their importance to the office's clinical functions has increased too. Keeping patients' charts on the computer is becoming more common. **Electronic medical records (EMR)** are gradually replacing paper charts.

EMR offers several advantages over traditional paper charts.

- Electronic records are easy to store and retrieve. The office will not run out of file space.
- Information is easy to add. Many systems use a touch screen to store a patient's vital signs and other information. Paper documents are scanned into the electronic chart.
- Charting is often better because it's readable and more complete. For example, the computer may require you to enter certain information before you can move to the next screen. This prevents missed documentation.
- Computer charting takes less time than writing notes in the chart by hand.

CREATING AND MAINTAINING A CHART

A medical office has a chart for each of its patients. One of your jobs will be to keep these records current. You'll do this by:

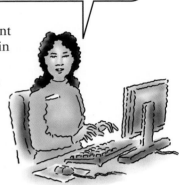

> Having electronic medical records (EMR) means a patient's file never gets misplaced.

- placing all correspondence, lab reports, and other medical information about the patient that arrives in the office in the proper location in the patient's chart
- making sure blank progress notes are always in the chart for the physician to use when the patient comes in for return visits

When a new patient makes an appointment, you will have to make a chart for that patient. The Hands On features on page 187 will tell you how to do this for both paper records and EMR.

How Charts Are Organized

Patients' charts are usually organized in one of two ways.

- The problem-oriented medical record (POMR) organizes information by the patient's problem. This is a good method for physicians who treat patients for a variety of problems.
- The source-oriented medical record (SOMR) files all items according to their source. For example, all lab reports are in one part of the chart, and all radiology results are in another.

Whichever method your office uses, one thing doesn't change. No matter what section of the chart a page is filed in, the most recent information always appears first in that section. In other words, you always place new pages on top of existing pages. This creates a reverse order to the information. The farther back you go in each section of a patient's chart, the older the information is.

POMR Organization. Family practices, pediatricians, and others who treat a variety of problems often this use this method of organizing charts. The patient's medical problems are listed on the first page of the chart. As each problem arises, it is added to the list and given a number.

All charting about that problem elsewhere in the chart is given the same number. When the problem no longer exists, that is recorded in the progress notes and an *X* is marked next to the problem on the problem list.

A POMR is divided into sections.

1. *Database.* The following information goes in this part of the chart:
   - the patient's chief complaint

- the present illness
- the patient's medical history
- review of systems
- physical examination
- lab reports

2. *Problem list.* This includes every past, present, and future problem the patient has that requires evaluation.

3. *Treatment plan.* This includes the workups, tests, and treatment each problem has required.

4. *Progress notes.* These are records of patient contacts that are numbered and grouped together. Some physicians may prefer to group these notes to relate to each numbered problem on the chart's problem list. Others might place them in chronological order.

SOMR Organization. Items in an SOMR are grouped by the type of item, not by the problem to which they're related. So, for example, all the x-ray reports are filed in one group, with the most recent report on top, and so on.

> Remember, items in a patient's chart are organized in reverse order. New information goes on top of the older information.

Each office's classification system may differ. But the major groupings in an SOMR generally include these:

- progress notes
- lab results
- radiography reports
- patient education

This approach to organizing charts is often used by specialists. It works because they don't treat a wide range of problems in the patients they see. But the SOMR is also the most common way charts are organized in all medical offices.

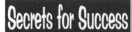

Secrets for Success | **CHART ORGANIZATION**

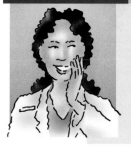

Here's a tip to help you recall the two main ways charts are organized.

- Remember that *P* stands for *problem*. In a POMR, records are organized around each medical *problem*.
- Remember that *S* stands for *source*. In an SOMR, records of the same type or *source*—such as x-ray results—are grouped together.

SOAP FORMAT

The SOAP format is one of the most common methods of documenting patient visits. The SOAP format is made up of four parts.

- The *subjective* part is the direct statement or description from the patient telling about his or her own condition. These notes should show the patient's exact words using actual quotations. For example, "I've been vomiting all night and have had diarrhea for the past two days. The last thing I was able to eat was crackers at dinner time last night."

- The *objective* part includes information the medical assistant and physician observe about the patient. It can include test results and vital signs. For example, "The patient appears weak, pale, and slightly dehydrated and has lost three pounds since her last visit."

- The *assessment* portion is a summary of the information from the first two parts. It is the preliminary patient diagnosis. If a diagnosis cannot be made yet, the provider lists possible disorders to be ruled out. For example, "Possible viral infection."

- The *plan* is a description of what should be done including any necessary diagnostic tests, treatments that will be given, and when the patient should follow up with the physician, if at all. For example, "Stool culture, CBC with diff, BRAT diet, and Imodium for the next 48 hours. Call office if symptoms worsen; return to office if patient not well by the end of the week."

No matter what form you use for documentation, always include the date, time, and your signature and credentials.

Forms

In some offices, the blank pages for charts are bought from an outside supplier. Other offices may create special forms to meet their needs more exactly. Additional forms, such as vaccination records, are required by federal law.

Progress Notes. A chart's progress notes record each contact with a patient—whether by phone, mail, e-mail, or in person—and briefly summarize what happened. Some offices use lined paper that has two columns. The date and time of the contact is written in the narrow left column, and the note is written on the lines in the right column. Other offices use plain or lined paper without columns for progress notes.

Medical History Forms. Medical offices use these types of forms to get medical and personal information from a new patient before she sees the physician. Many offices mail these forms to patients before their first appointment. The patient then brings the completed form to the appointment. This process has several advantages.

- The patient has time to think carefully about and answer the questions.

- The patient can gather information about the family medical history.

- The medical office receives a more accurate and complete patient medical history.

In an EMR, the information from this form is keyed or scanned into the patient's chart. The completed form is then shredded to protect the privacy of the patient's information.

> In an electronic system, paper documents are scanned into the patient's chart. Then, the papers are shredded.

Flow Sheets. A flow sheet is a form that allows information to be recorded in a table or on a graph. An office may use several types of flow sheets. They are generally designed for a specific use, such as charting vital signs or tracking prescribed medications. They are also often color-coded. The graph on which to record a child's height and weight at each visit might be printed on pink paper, for example.

Flow sheets are very useful forms to have in a chart. Here are some reasons why.

- They limit the need for long, handwritten notes containing the information.

- They eliminate the need to search through pages of the chart to find the information.

- They give you all the information at once. This makes it easier to spot any changes over time.

You can see an example of a medications flow sheet, reduced from its actual size, on page 172. In an EMR, the software can create the flow sheet. All you have to do is enter the information. The computer automatically puts it on the graph or table.

Ardmore Family Practice, P.A.
2805 Lyndhurst Avenue
Winston-Salem, NC 27103
PHONE: 336-659-0076
FAX: 336-659-0272

Patient: MICHAEL FIELDS

Date: 02-12-2007 9:06 AM

MEDICATIONS

Date	Drug Name	Strength/Form	Dispense	Refill	Sig	Last Dose/ Disc Date	Status
1/28/07	SINGULAIR	10 MG TABS	5	0	1 PO BID		NEW
1/28/07	ZITHROMAX	200 MG/5ML SUSR	5	0	1 PO Q DAY		NEW
1/22/07	ACCUPRIL	10 MG TABS	34	4	1 PO QD	1/28/07	CONTINUE
1/22/07	ADVIL	200 MG TABS	1	1	1/2 Q A.M.	1/25/07	NEW
1/22/07	ALTACE	5 MG CAPS	60	5	ONE TWICE DAILY	1/28/07	CONTINUE
1/22/07	MACROBID	100 MG CAPS	14	0	1 PO BID	1/28/07	CONTINUE
8/26/06	ALTACE	5 MG CAPS	60	5	ONE TWICE DAILY		CONTINUE
8/7/06	PRECOSE	25 MG CAPS	60	0	1/2 B.I.D.	10/5/06	NEW
5/2/05	ACCUPRIL	10 MG TABS	34	4	1 PO QD		NEW
5/2/05	ACCUPRIL	20 MG TABS	30	0	1 PO QD		NEW
5/2/05	ACCUPRIL	40 MG TABS	30	5	1 PO QD		NEW
4/25/05	ACCUPRIL	20 MG TABS	30	0	1 PO QD	4/25/05	NEW
4/25/05	ACCUPRIL	40 MG TABS	30	5	1 PO QD		NEW
4/25/05	MACROBID	100 MG TABS	14	0	1 PO BID	5/1/05	NEW
3/2/05	ACIPHEX 20 MG	TABS	30	6	1 PO QD		NEW
3/2/05	ACTOS 30 MG	TABS	30	2	1 PO QD		NEW
1/23/05	ENTEX PSE	120-600 MG TB12	45	0	1 PO BID		NEW
1/23/05	NASONEX	50 MCG/ACT SUSP	1	3	2 SPRAYS EACH NOSTRIL QD		NEW
8/24/03	ADALAT CC	60 MG TBCR	34	5	1 PO QD	8/24/03	NEW
7/8/03	NITROGLYCERIN	0.4 MG/DOSE AERS	100	1	1 TAB SL Q 5 MIN X 3, IF CHEST PAIN PERS	7/8/03	NEW
6/26/03	CLARITIN	10 MG TABS	30	5	ONE EVERY MORNING		NEW
6/23/03	CELEBREX 100 MG	CAPS	90	3	1 PO Q AM AND 2 PO Q PM		NEW
6/3/03	GLUCOPHAGE	850 MG TABS	90	6	ONE 3 TIMES DAILY	6/3/03	NEW
6/3/03	HYTRIN	5 MG CAPS	30	6	ONE EVERY DAY	6/3/03	NEW

Maintaining Charts

A huge amount of paperwork comes into the typical medical office each day. This includes:

- x-ray reports
- blood test results
- other test results
- hospital records
- notes from other physicians
- insurance information

All this material must be sorted and put in the proper place in the right patient's chart. In many offices, the medical assistant has this responsibility. It's an important one. An office can't run smoothly and efficiently if information on a patient isn't dealt with correctly. The Hands On feature on page 188 contains a step-by-step procedure for adding this material to a patient's charts.

Holding. Documents that have been reviewed by the physician should be filed in patients' charts daily. It's important that you do not let unfiled test results and other records pile up. This information needs to be in patients' charts where it can help the physician in treating them.

Closer Look   RECORDS FOR FILING

Facilities that perform diagnostic tests on your patients are required to produce a report of their findings. They send these reports to your office to be filed in the patients' charts. Here are some other types of records that often must be added to the charts.

- reports of minor surgical procedures
- consultation reports from other physicians
- history and physical examination (H&P) reports

Many physicians dictate their H&Ps on patients into a handheld recorder. An office employee or outside service later transcribes these recordings—that is, puts them into print form. The medical assistant must then add these records to patients' charts. Sometimes, physicians' progress notes will be dictated and transcribed too. These notes also must be filed in the charts.

Until documents are filed, they should be held in a specific place in the office. This allows staff to find the records if they need the information before the records are filed. This holding area should be used only until the daily filing can be done.

Shingling. Most lab reports are produced by computer. They come ready to be filed in patients' charts. Any report or other document that is smaller than a full-size sheet of paper must be attached to a full-size sheet of paper before being put in the proper place in the chart. Some examples of these smaller documents could include phone message slips or urinalysis slips that don't take up a full page.

Sometimes several lab results are attached to the same sheet of paper in a process known as *shingling*. The process gets this name because the page of reports looks like shingles on a roof. This is how you shingle documents in a patient's medical record.

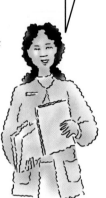

Before you add items to a patient's chart, have the physician read and initial them first.

- Tape the first document across its top near the bottom of a full-size piece of paper. Make sure the bottom edges of both sheets of paper are lined up.

- Each document is added over the previous one with a piece of tape across its top.

- Each sheet can then be lifted to view the one beneath it.

Closer Look CONDITIONING

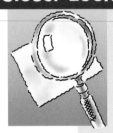

Some items require "conditioning" before they are placed in a patient's file. Here's how to condition documents.

- Remove all staples and paper clips. Over time, these will cause the corners of the chart to bulge if they are left in place. Paper clips also may accidentally attach to other papers. Staples left in a file could cause injury.

- Make sure the patient's name is on each piece of paper. This is important in case an unattached second page ever gets separated from the first page of a document.

- Mend any tears in documents with tape.

- Attach any small documents to a piece of full-size paper before putting it in the chart.

WORKERS' COMPENSATION RECORDS

From time to time, a current patient will seek treatment for an injury or illness he got on the job. Do not add these treatment records to the patient's chart.

If this is a workers' compensation case, you must create new separate medical and financial records for the patient. **Workers' compensation** is health insurance the law requires employers to have for workers who suffer job-related injuries.

Unless the injury is life threatening, you must first have approval from the patient's employer to treat the patient and bill for workers' compensation. (You'll read more about getting this approval in Chapter 8.) Be sure to write the name of the person who authorizes treatment in the patient's new medical record. Also chart any additional information you receive that relates to the approval process.

A workers' compensation chart belongs to the patient's employer. The employer's workers' compensation insurer can review the information in this record, even if the patient opposes it. But you should not give any information about the patient's other health conditions, or from his other chart, to the employer's insurer.

Workers' compensation cases are kept open for two years after the last date the patient was treated for the injury or illness. This is in case any follow-up care is needed. Even after care is complete, keep the record separate from the patient's other chart. But you may add information from the workers' compensation chart to the patient's other chart if the need arises.

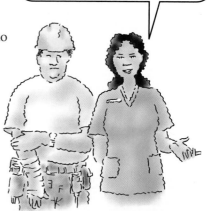

Remember, don't file treatment records for workers' compensation injuries in the patient's regular chart.

Making Entries in Medical Records

A patient's medical record is a legal document. It can be presented in court as evidence in a malpractice suit. The entries the office staff makes in a chart can help win a lawsuit—or prevent one altogether—if they are:

- accurate and complete
- legible, or clear enough to be read easily
- timely, that is, written at the time of the event

On the other hand, if charting is messy, inaccurate, or improperly done, it can raise questions about what actually happened. This might cause a health care provider to lose a malpractice suit.

SAMPLE CHART ENTRIES

Which of these entries explaining a canceled appointment would be a better defense in a malpractice suit?

- *9-15-05: Pt. called to Cx appt for recheck of UTI on 9-16. Says she is feeling better. Advised to keep appt since Dr. Smith wants to repeat UA to see if her bladder infection has cleared up. Pt. states, "I don't see any need for that. I'm not coming." Dr. Smith was advised.*
  _____ *Fred Lane, MA*

- *9-15-05: Pt. called to Cx appt.*
  _____ *Fred Lane, MA*

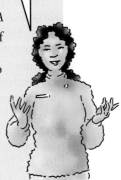

Documenting, <u>documentation</u>, and <u>charting</u> are professional terms that mean writing something in a patient's chart.

Did you choose the first note? The golden rule of charting is if it's not documented, it didn't happen. Therefore, the second note would be absolutely no help in a lawsuit over this patient's bladder infection. All patient procedures, assessments, evaluations, teaching, and communications must be properly documented. The Hands On feature on page 188 provides guidelines to help make your charting appropriate.

Closer Look | THE NARRATIVE FORMAT

Most of your writing in charts will be in narrative form. This is the oldest and least structured style of charting. It's just a short statement that tells of the contact with the patient, what happened, and the outcome. Here are some examples of narrative charting.

10/17/05: Pt. called C/o fever, sore throat. Asked to speak to Dr. Johnson. Told pt. to come in, explained that Dr. can't treat her over phone. Given appt for tomorrow at 10:00 A.M.
_____ *Jennifer Wise, CMA*
10/18/05: Pt called and stated that she felt "90% better."
Appt Cx. _____ *Jennifer Wise, CMA*

Closer Look — THE NARRATIVE FORMAT (*continued*)

12/16/05: Lab work normal. Called pt. per Dr. Johnson and told her to notify us if her fever is not gone tomorrow. Pt. states, "I guess I feel somewhat better." Pt. will call office p.r.n.
_____ *Jennifer Wise, CMA*

Notice that each entry contains the name and credentials of the person who wrote it. It is important to include both. Experts say to use your full name rather than your initials.

DOCUMENTING PATIENT CONTACTS

Besides appointments, your medical office will have other contacts with patients. These must all be documented in the patient's chart. Most offices do this in the progress notes. Some may have a special form or log on which to record communications with patients.

All actions taken by the physician—or by staff at the physician's direction—must be documented in the patient's chart. Here are some examples.

Legal Brief — THE MEDICAL RECORD AS A LEGAL DOCUMENT

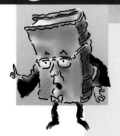

It's common to see abbreviations in charting entries. Using them saves writing time and space. Your office should have a list of standard abbreviations. The table on the next page shows some abbreviations that are used commonly in charting.

Be careful how you use abbreviations. Errors in patient care could result if you use a wrong abbreviation, or one that has an unclear meaning, in the chart, For example, if you write "BS normal" in a chart, do you mean bowel sounds or breath sounds? What about blood sugar? To someone reading the chart, *BS* could stand for any of the three.

Also, always use the standard abbreviations instead of making up your own. Remember, following these procedures is vital because the medical record is a legal document.

Abbreviations Used in Charting

Abbreviation	Meaning	Abbreviation	Meaning	Abbreviation	Meaning
ā	Before	Fx	Fracture	q.i.d.	Four times a day
abd	Abdomen	h.s.	Bedtime (hour of sleep)	R	Right
ant.	Anterior	Hx	History	R/O	Rule out
AP	Anteroposterior	L	Left	RLE	Right lower extremity
appt	Appointment	LLE	Left lower extremity	RLQ	Right lower quadrant
Ax	Axillary	LLQ	Left lower quadrant	RUE	Right upper extremity
b.i.d.	Twice a day	LUE	Left upper extremity	RUQ	Right upper quadrant
BP	Blood pressure	LUQ	Left upper quadrant	R/s	Rescheduled
c̄	With	NKDA	No known drug allergies	s̄	Without
CC	Chief complaint	noct.	Nocturnal	SOB	Shortness of breath
c/o	Complains of	p̄	After	spec	Specimen
CPE, CPX	Complete physical exam	p.c.	After a meal	s/p	After (status post)
Cx	Cancelled	PE	Physical examination	STAT	Immediately
D/C	Discontinue	p.r.n.	As needed	t.i.d.	Three times a day
F	Fahrenheit	pt.	Patient	TPR	Temperature, pulse, respiration

- When you phone a prescription to the pharmacy, record your action in the patient's chart.
- If the physician tells you to call the patient with some test results, write this communication in the chart.

Timely Charting

As you already know, the pages in a chart are in reverse order, with the most recent page on top. The notes on each page, however, should be in **chronological order.** This means the *earliest* entry should be at the top of the page. Entries with more recent dates should be in order down the page.

Dates that are out of order and gaps between entries may confuse the reader. They also make the office appear to be disorganized. This is one reason why you should record contacts with patients soon after they take place. Another reason is the events will still be fresh in your mind. If you wait, someone might write another, later event on the page first. Also, you might forget the details of the encounter.

Charting Communications from Patients

Phone calls from patients are usually charted in **narrative** style. (See the Closer Look on The Narrative Format on page 176.) Document the conversation immediately. Include the following information in your note:

- the date and time of the call
- what the patient requested or said
- what you said and the actions you took

If your office uses special patient communication forms, you should attach the form to the progress notes when you chart the call.

E-mails from patients should be printed out and placed in the chart. Any replies also should be printed out and included with the progress notes.

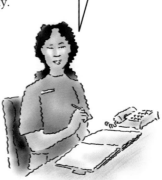

> For timely and accurate charting, promptly document all contacts with patients.

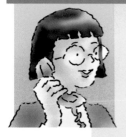

Ask the Professional CORRECTING ERRORS

Q: *I made a mistake while writing in a patient's chart the other day. I got an ink eraser out of my desk to correct my mistake. The office nurse saw me and told me to stop. She said I needed to learn how to make a correction properly. What's wrong with the way I was doing it? And what's the right way to make a correction?*

A: As you already know, a patient's chart is a legal document. That's why everything you write in it must be in ink. It's also why when you make a writing error, it's critical that you correct it properly.

You should never write over, scribble out, use white-out, or attempt to erase information in a medical record. Those kinds of corrections could be seen as attempts to cover something up. Instead, when you make an error, follow these steps.

- Draw a single line through the incorrect information.
- Write the word *error* and then the correct information.
- Initial the correction and date it.

In an electronic record, you can click on an icon to make a correction. The original information will not be deleted. As a further safeguard, some computer charting software only allows certain users to change information after it's been saved.

Managing Medical Records

Good management of an office's paper medical records requires five basic things.

1. Properly and accurately create the charts of new patients. The Hands On feature about creating paper charts on page 187 gives you step-by-step guidance on how to do this.

2. File new items in patients' charts accurately and in a timely manner. This task is covered in the Hands On feature on page 188.

3. Properly and accurately retrieve and return patient's charts to the office's medical records files. Doing this requires understanding and following one of the filing systems you will read about next.

4. Repair and replace folders, labels, and stickers. Handling the charts of frequently seen patients over and over will cause these charts to wear out. All charts must be kept in good condition.

5. Remove and store the charts of patients who have not been seen for a long time. You will read more about this topic later in this chapter.

FILING SYSTEMS

The two main systems used to file and retrieve medical records are:

- the alphabetical filing system
- numeric (number) filing systems

Some offices use both systems for different types of files. Also, there are two ways of filing medical records by number.

Alphabetic Filing

This method of organizing medical records places them in alphabetical order by patients' last names. If two or more patients have the same last name, the system orders them alphabetically by their first names, and so on. The Hands On feature on page 190 gives you step-by-step guidelines for filing records this way.

Some offices also use color coding with alphabetical files. A color-coded bar is placed next to the label with the patient's name. The color of the bar depends on the letter of the alphabet. For example, patients whose last names begin with the letters *A* to *F* might have blue bars on their charts; *G* to *L*, green bars; *M* to *T*, yellow bars, and so on.

This color-coded system makes it easier to find misplaced charts. With one glance at a file cabinet, for example, you could spot a green tab in the middle of the yellow ones.

Numeric Filing

Numeric systems usually assign a six-digit number to each patient. Patient charts are then filed in numerical order. The

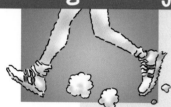

Running Smoothly   OUT GUIDES

What can you do to spend less time refiling patients' charts?

Each day's appointments leave you dozens of patients' charts to be returned to the office's medical records files. If you could perform this task more efficiently, you would have more time for your other duties.

Here's a way to refile charts more quickly—and more accurately too! Use out guides. These are plastic or cardboard sheets with a tab labeled OUT GUIDE at the end and a pocket on the side. A special card goes in this pocket.

- Before you remove a patient's chart from the files, write the patient's name on an out guide card. Also, write the date, your initials, and where the chart will be located.

- Put the card in the pocket of an out guide.

- When you remove the patient's chart from the files, put the out guide in its place. This tells anyone who comes looking for the chart later where it can be found.

- When you refile the chart, look for the out guide in the right area of the files.

- Compare the name on the chart with the name on the out guide card. If they are the same, put the chart back in the files in that location.

- Remove the out guide from the files. Also, remove the card from the out guide so both can be used again.

As you can see, using out guides can help you find a chart that's been removed from the files too.

> Using out guides makes your filing tasks easier, faster, and more efficient.

digits are usually run together when the label is put on the chart. But they are read as three groups of two digits each. For example, patient number 324478 is read as 32 44 78. When you organize charts this way, it's called **straight digit filing.** That's because you are reading the number straight out, from left to right.

Another type of numeric filing is **terminal digit filing.** The label will look the same in this way of filing—324478. But it will be read and filed in reverse order, from right to left: 78 44 32.

Numeric filing systems have a couple of advantages over the alphabetical system.

- It makes no difference if two or more patients have the same name, such as John Smith. Each John Smith will have a different number on his chart and records. Their charts probably will be in different places in the files. It's harder for their charts—or the records that are filed in them—to be mixed up.
- The results of tests for HIV and AIDS are strictly confidential. Using numbers instead of names to identify charts and the records in them gives patients added privacy. This feature has helped make numeric filing systems more popular.

Numeric filing systems require you to keep what's called a master patient index in a secure location. This list is a **cross-reference** of all patient names and patient numbers.

- Finding a patient's name on the alphabetical part of the list will give you the patient's number.
- Finding a record's number on the numerical list will tell you which patient the record belongs.

When patients come in for appointments, you must look up their names on the master patient index and get their number codes. Only then will you be able to find and pull their charts for their appointments.

On the other hand, there's no need to know patients' names in order to add items to their charts. You'll find charts and file items in them by numbers. This is one of the ways numeric systems help protect patient privacy. You can't tell just by looking at a test result, for example, to which patient the result belongs.

Other Filing Systems

Your office will have more files than just patient charts. Some examples of other records it might keep are:

- employee personnel files
- inventories of equipment and supplies

Closer Look   NUMERIC FILING SYSTEMS

Here's an example of how straight digit filing and terminal digit filing work. Suppose these records are to be filed numerically:

Curtis, Ralph	334387
Ford, LeRoy	213456
King, Cathy	321138
Moore, Sharon	979779

In a straight-digit filing system, the proper order is:

Ford, LeRoy	213456
King, Cathy	321138
Curtis, Ralph	334387
Moore, Sharon	979779

In a terminal-digit filing system, the proper order is:

King, Cathy	321138
Ford, LeRoy	213456
Moore, Sharon	979779
Curtis, Ralph	334387

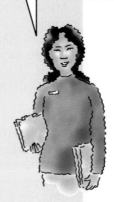

If your office uses more than one filing system, be careful not to mix up the charts. Using different color folders for each system can prevent errors.

- records of past supply orders
- accounts payable
- insurance records
- catalogs from suppliers

Your office might use a system of **subject filing** for keeping such records. This is a system in which records are grouped alphabetically according to their subject—insurance, medications, referrals, and so on. Here are some other filing systems you might see or use.

- *Geographic filing.* Documents are grouped alphabetically according to location, such as state, county, or city.

- *Chronological filing.* Documents are grouped in the order of their date, such as year or month.

Chart Maintenance

Over the years, the charts of longtime patients may become worn. As you are removing or returning charts to the medical records files, keep an eye out for labels or stickers that are peeling and folders that are worn out. You should replace these before a folder tears or a label or sticker falls off. Some patients' charts may become so large that a second folder must be created. Be sure to clearly mark the new folder as "Volume 2."

CLASSIFYING MEDICAL RECORDS

Patients' charts are classified in three categories.

- active records
- inactive records
- closed records

Active Records

Active records are the charts of patients who have been seen within the past few years. The exact amount of time varies from office to office. For most offices, it's between one and five years.

Store the charts of active patients in places that are easy to access. These are the charts you will be retrieving, using, and refiling the most.

Inactive Records

Inactive records are the charts of patients who have not been seen within the time limit the office sets for active patients. They haven't used the physician's services during that period. But they have not terminated the contract with the physician formally. (You read about contracts and contract termination in Chapter 2.) Also, no one has told the office the patients have moved, found another physician, or died.

You should keep the charts of inactive patients in the office, although they don't have to be as easy to access as the active charts. Many offices store inactive charts on the bottom shelves of the medical records files. Doing this reduces the need for bending to find or refile the charts of active patients.

Closed Records

Closed records are the charts of patients who have ended their relationship with the physician. Here are the main reasons you would classify a patient's chart as closed.

- The patient has moved away.
- The physician-patient relationship has been terminated by letter.
- The patient needs no further treatment from the physician.
- The patient has died.

Closed records should be removed from the files and stored.

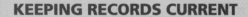

Running Smoothly

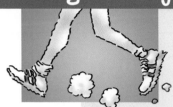

KEEPING RECORDS CURRENT

How do you identify and remove the charts of inactive patients from the active records files?

The Hands On feature on page 187 tells you to put a year label on the folder when you create a chart for a new patient. Taking this step allows you to keep the active charts in the files separate from the inactive ones. Here's how.

- Each time an established patient visits the office, check the year label on his chart.

- If the year label is not for the current year, replace it with the current year's label.

- At the end of each year, go through the medical records and remove the charts of all patients whose year labels are older than the limit the office sets for active patients. For example, if the office requires that a patient must have been seen within the past year to remain active, you would remove all charts that don't have this year's label on them. Since you put new labels on the charts of all patients who came in during the year, none of their charts will be removed.

- If the office sets a five-year time limit for active patients, you would remove all charts from the active files that have year labels more than five years old. Some offices might set a three-year time limit. Always check your office's policy before removing any charts.

Record Retention

All patient charts should be kept permanently, but they don't all need to be kept in the office. Closed records and old inactive records can be stored somewhere else. They also can be put on microfilm or microfiche. This method involves photographing each page and storing it in reduced form on a roll of film or on a small card. Old records might even be scanned into a computer and stored on its hard drive. Records also are stored on CDs or DVDs to avoid taking up space on the hard drive.

You read about the statute of limitations in Chapter 2. This is the time limit for filing a lawsuit for wrongdoing. It varies from state to state. But in some states, malpractice suits can be filed up to two years after the possible malpractice is discovered. Also, if the patient was a minor, the time limit may not even begin until he or she becomes an adult. These are the main reasons old charts should be stored permanently.

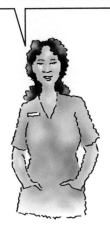

Never throw away a patient's medical record, even if the record is closed. All patient records should be kept permanently, regardless of where those records are filed.

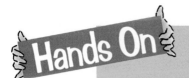

CREATING A PATIENT'S PAPER CHART

5-1

A medical record must be created for all new patients before the physician sees them for the first time. Follow these steps to create a paper chart.

1. Type the patient's name on a label and apply it to an appropriate place on the chart.
   - Type the patient's name in unit order—last name first, followed by first name, and middle initial. For example, type *Smith, John L.*, not *John L. Smith*.

2. Apply the alphabetical, color, or numerical label to the appropriate place on the chart. These labels help make filing and retrieval easier.

3. Add the year label to the appropriate place on the chart. Having this label makes it easier to find and remove inactive charts from the files.

4. Place the appropriate stickers on the outside of the chart. Depending on office policy, these may include:
   - an allergy sticker with the patient's allergies listed on it
   - an advance directive sticker noting whether the patient has a living will or power of attorney (POA) for health care
   - a label with insurance information

5. Insert the dividers and add the appropriate paperwork to the correct side and section of the chart. This paperwork may include:
   - the patient's personal and insurance information
   - the patient's completed medical history form
   - blank progress notes for the physician's first encounter with the patient
   - any past medical records on the patient that are available
   - a copy of the patient's living will or POA for health care (if any)

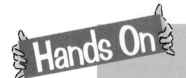

CREATING A PATIENT'S ELECTRONIC CHART

5-2

A medical record, or chart, must be created for all new patients. Follow these steps to create an electronic medical record (EMR).

1. Enter the patient information into the computer using your office's electronic charting software.

2. Scan into the patient's computer file any paper records that already exist. These may include:
   - the personal information form completed by the patient
   - the medical history form completed by the patient
   - any past medical records on the patient that are available
   - a copy of the patient's living will or POA for health care (if any)

3. Dispose of scanned paper records according to your office's policy.

ADDING ITEMS TO A PATIENT'S CHART

5-3

If you follow these steps to add information in patients' charts, both the charts and the task will be organized.

1. Divide the papers to be filed into groups according to each patient's name. (Use the same procedure as in the Hands On feature for Filing Charts on page 190 to sort papers.)

2. Make sure the patient's name is on each page of the papers in his or her group. Also make sure the papers contain the doctor's initials and date.
   - Write the name in the upper right corner if it is missing.
   - Remove any staples or paper clips from the pages.

3. Mend any torn pages with tape.

4. Tape small items to standard-size pieces of paper.

5. Add each item to the correct section of the chart using the office's organization system. Add items in reverse chronological order, with the most recent item in each section on top.

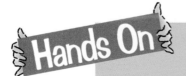

CHARTING IN A PATIENT'S MEDICAL RECORD 5-4

Make sure you know the office policy for charting. Find out who is allowed to write in patient charts. If you are expected to document patient contacts, follow these guidelines.

1. Make sure you have the correct chart. Use the patient's birth date as a double check, especially if the patient has a common name.

2. Always document in ink.
   - Use dark ink. Black ink shows up best on photocopies.
   - Write your full name and credentials at the end of each entry.

3. Always record the date of each entry. Some offices also record the time of the entry. Indicate A.M. or P.M. or use military time.

4. Print legibly. Printing is easier to read than cursive writing.

5. Check spelling, especially the spelling of medical terms, before you write them in the chart.

6. Use only abbreviations that are accepted by your office. Abbreviations can cause confusion if they are open to interpretation or are used incorrectly.

7. Document as soon as possible after completing a task. This practice will promote accuracy.

8. When charting a patient's statements, use quotation marks to show the patient's own words.

9. Don't try to diagnose. If the patient says, "My throat is sore," don't write *pharyngitis*. It's not within the scope of your training to diagnose.

10. Always document these events in the chart:
    - all phone conversations with the patient
    - attempts to remind patients of their appointments
    - missed appointments and your follow-up actions

11. Never chart false information. Be honest. For example, if you gave a wrong medication or performed a wrong procedure, document it as soon as you've reported it to a supervisor. State only the facts. Don't draw any conclusions or place blame.

12. Never chart for someone else or let someone else chart for you.

Hands On

FILING CHARTS ALPHABETICALLY

5-5

Follow these guidelines to file patients' medical records properly in an alphabetic system. These procedures also apply to sorting documents to be added to patients' charts in an alphabetic filing system.

1. File according to last name, then first name, then middle initial.

2. Treat each letter in a name as a separate unit.

3. Treat letters that are by themselves as separate units. For example, in filing C. B. Hill's chart, *Hill* would be the first unit, *C.* the second unit, and *B.* the third unit.

4. Treat hyphenated names as one name. For example, Sally P. Smith-Jones should be filed as *Smith-Jones, Sally P.*, not as *Jones, Sally P. Smith.*

5. File abbreviated names as if they were spelled out. For example, file Wm. Miller as *Miller, William* and file Mary St. James as *Saint James, Mary.*

6. Last names beginning with *Mac* and *Mc* can be filed together or in regular alphabetical order, depending on the policy of your office.

7. *Jr.* and *Sr.* should be used in labeling and filing patients' records. Treat them as a fourth unit and file them alphabetically. (Using this rule, *Jr.* would come before *Sr.*)

8. Professional titles and initials are placed after a name and are not included in the filing system. Thus, Dr. Joe P. Jacobs, M.D., would be filed as *Jacobs, Joe P., M.D.*

9. If two or more patients' last, first, and middle names or initials are identical, use their birth dates to determine the order of their charts. Typically, the patient with the most recent birth date would come first. However, it's important to check with your office's policy.

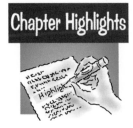

Chapter Highlights

- Patient charts are legal records that show the quality of patient care.
- Preparing and maintaining patient charts is an important responsibility.
- Understanding chart organization is important—in order to file items in charts properly and to write in charts correctly.
- All patients' contact with the office must be documented properly.
- Medical records files can be organized alphabetically or numerically.
- Charts are grouped into active, inactive, and closed categories.
- Computer technology is changing the way medical records are organized, maintained, and stored.

Chapter 6

MANAGING FINANCES

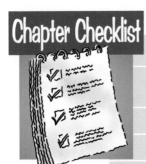

Chapter Checklist

- Explain fee schedules and describe the main forms of payment
- Summarize the process of identifying and collecting unpaid bills
- Perform billing and collection procedures
- Explain the importance and use of the day sheet
- Post entries on a day sheet
- Summarize the manual system for managing patients' accounts
- Describe the functions of a computer accounting system
- Perform accounts receivable procedures
- Post adjustments
- Process credit balance
- Post NSF checks
- Post collection agency payments
- Process refunds
- Describe how medical offices use bank services
- Prepare a bank deposit
- Identify accounts payable functions and relate how they are handled

A medical office is a business with two main goals. One is to help people keep or regain good health. The other is to make money. These two goals go hand in hand. A medical office must make money if it is to keep serving patients' needs. This means charging fees for the care it provides. Without these fees, it won't have the money it needs to continue offering services.

To succeed financially, a medical office also must maintain patients' accounts, collect the fees it charges, and manage office expenses and payroll. You'll learn about these basic tasks in this chapter, as well as about fee schedules, bookkeeping, and other financial aspects of the health care business.

Setting and Collecting Fees

The fees most offices charge for office visits, lab work, and other procedures and treatments are based on several factors. One of these is the cost of running the office. Some of these expenses include:

- office or building rent
- utilities (heat, light, water, phone, etc.)
- employees' wages
- equipment and supplies
- insurance (especially malpractice insurance)

The principles of RBRVS and UCR guide how an office structures its fees. RBRVS stands for "resource-based relative value scale." This guideline measures the relative value of a service. It does so by comparing a service to other services, considering their difficulty, the time required, and so on.

UCR stands for "usual, customary, and reasonable." Here's what goes into calculating UCR fees.

- usual—the average fee the physician has charged for the service over a period of time
- customary—the average fee that other physicians in the geographic area charge for the service
- reasonable—the fee that meets the criteria of the usual and customary fees. Reimbursement is based on the lower of the two fees.

You'll learn more about RBRVS and UCR in Chapters 7 and 8 when you read about coding medical procedures and billing patients' health insurance.

FEE SCHEDULES

A **fee schedule** is a list of accepted charges for specific medical procedures. A medical practice can have more than one fee schedule unless state laws restrict this practice. Because health plans have different ways of calculating UCR charges—and thus what they'll pay—some offices may follow several fee schedules for the same set of services. There might be another fee schedule for patients who are **private pay**—that is, paying the bill with no help from insurance. Medicare, Medicaid, and workers' compensation companies also have fee schedules.

It's not unusual for a medical office to have numerous fee schedules. It's suggested, however, that providers have only one fee schedule that applies to all carriers to make sure there are no violations.

In addition, many physicians are preferred providers or **participating providers.**

- *Preferred providers* are health care providers that are part of a health plan's network. You first read about them in Chapter 4. Preferred providers have agreed to provide services to the health plan's members for a reduced fee.
- *Participating providers* are those who have joined a managed-care organization. These organizations are designed to help control the high costs of health care. You will learn more about managed care in Chapter 8.

Medical offices become preferred providers or participating providers to increase their number of patients. In return, they agree to accept what the plan pays for services.

Discussing Fees in Advance

It's a good idea to discuss fees before treatment begins. Patients need to know in advance whether the office is a preferred provider or participating provider with their health plan.

One way to begin this discussion is by giving the patient an office brochure to read. The brochure should contain not only the office's phone number and hours, but also its policies on payment. This information should include:

- policies about credit and collections
- policies for insurance billing
- policies regarding patient co-payments

Patients with managed-care plans and many other health plans are required to pay a **co-pay.** This is an amount the plan sets as the patient's share of the bill. You should collect the co-pay at the time of service. This policy should be stated clearly in the office brochure. Many offices also post a sign in the waiting area that co-pays are due at the time of the appointment.

Some offices will have different rules that will apply in specific situations. When working with self-pay patients who don't have insurance, always try to collect the entire amount they owe. If this is not possible, ask to see a picture ID, such as a driver's license. Photocopy this ID for the patient's account file.

> Most insurance companies require that you bill the company before billing the patient. But be sure to collect the patient's co-pay at the time of the visit.

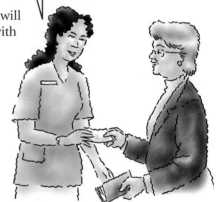

Forms of Payment

A patient usually can pay for services in a medical office in one of three ways.

- *Cash.* Many patients will request a receipt to keep for their own records.
- *Personal check.* If a new patient pays by check, get two forms of identification.
- *Credit card.* This is the best way to be paid, even though the credit card company charges the office a fee.

More and more medical offices welcome credit cards. Some even accept debit cards too. This convenience is expensive. The card company usually charges the office 1.8% of the patient's payment. But paying this charge is often less costly than billing the patient and getting the money a month later—or maybe not at all!

Insurance Payments. The insurance companies pay the largest amount of money for services. For this reason, it's critical that you keep patients' insurance information up to date. Many offices ask for a patient's health insurance card at each visit. That way, any changes in insurance coverage can be noted and recorded in the patient's account.

> Always copy both sides of a patient's insurance card. Place the photocopy of the card and the driver's license either on the right or the left side of the chart under the patient information sheet.

Adjusting Fees

Sometimes, you'll have to make **adjustments** (changes in the fees charged) to a patient's account. This will occur when your office receives a payment from an insurance company that you are contracted with.

They will tell you what the allowed amount is and you will then have to adjust or write off the difference.

You will bill out the normal fee to the insurance company, even if the office is required by the contract to charge a lower fee. When the insurance payment is received, it will include an explanation of benefits (EOB). Once the EOB is received, you'll know how much the insurance company allows, how much to write off, and how much you can bill the patient.

The EOB will tell you how much you can collect for the service. You must then credit the patient's account for the difference between what the office charged and what the insurance company allowed. Once the credit adjustment is made, you can bill the patient if any unpaid balance remains due. You will learn more about how to do these things later in this chapter.

Professional Courtesy. Professional courtesy is when a provider treats another health care professional for free or for a reduced fee. Here again, you must charge the normal fee, and then do a credit adjustment for the amount of the discount. You can write "professional courtesy" in the description column of the patient's account record.

When dealing with professional courtesy, keep in mind that it changes how you bill the insurance company, if at all. If you bill the insurance company, you must bill for the same reduced fee that you charged the patient. Billing the insurance company for the full amount could involve your office in insurance fraud.

Giving Patients Credit

Depending on the treatment provided, health care costs can be very high. It's not always easy for patients to pay their bill—even a balance remaining after insurance has paid. Some offices extend patients **credit,** or permission to pay later. They allow patients to pay the amount due over time on a monthly payment plan.

Experts estimate that it costs about $8 a month to bill a patient. The following expenses are involved:

- office supplies, including envelopes, the paper on which the bills are printed, and printer ink
- employees' wages for the time it takes to prepare and mail monthly statements
- postage costs

Because of these expenses, some offices charge patients interest on their monthly accounts. Adding a 1 or 1.5 percent charge, for example, to a patient's unpaid balance each month helps the office recover the costs of sending out bills.

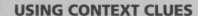

Secrets for Success — USING CONTEXT CLUES

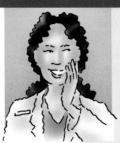

Many words have more than one meaning. Take the word *credit*, for instance. It has been used already in at least two ways in this chapter:

- You read that you should *credit* a patient's account when an insurance payment is for less than the amount billed.
- You read that some offices offer *credit* to patients who can't pay their entire bill.

A word's context—or the words that come before and after it—often provides clues to what the word means. For example, the first sentence suggests that *credit* means "to add something to the patient's account." The context of the second sentence suggests that in this case *credit* means "payment over time."

Here's yet another meaning for *credit*.

- "She deserves a lot of credit for working hard to become a medical assistant."

What do you think *credit* means in this case? If you said *praise*, you have correctly applied the context clues to the way the word was used.

The physician or office manager usually decides whether or not to allow a patient to pay his bill over time. In a large office, the business manager might make this decision. Typically, as a medical assistant, you will not be authorized to make credit arrangements with patients by yourself.

Monthly Billing

You should send all patients who have an unpaid balance a bill each month. This applies to those whose insurance plan didn't cover all their charges, as well as to patients who have made credit arrangements to pay over time.

Each patient's bill should show all changes in the account since the last bill. These changes might include:

- charges for any new visits and treatments
- payments received from insurance plans
- payments received from the patient
- insurance discounts or other adjustments to the account

Legal Brief — EXTENDING CREDIT

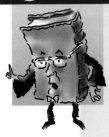

State and federal laws control the extension of credit. Here are some points to keep in mind.

- Credit can't be denied because of someone's gender, race or nationality, age, marital status, religion, or source of income. In general, this means that if you give one patient credit, you can't refuse another patient the same terms.

- If your office charges interest on monthly accounts, the law requires that patients be given a truth-in-lending statement. This notice tells patients the interest rate and any other costs they incur if they pay their bill over time.

- Different states have different laws about extending credit. Some states have laws limiting the amount of interest that can be charged.

If the patient has received credit and is making monthly payments, the bill should show any interest charged. It should show the amount of the next scheduled payment as well.

All bills should clearly show the total unpaid balance that remains due. This allows the patient to pay more than her scheduled monthly payment, if desired, or even to pay off the balance in full. The Hands On procedure on page 224 offers further specific guidance for preparing and sending bills.

BILLING CYCLES

Larger offices have many bills they need to send each month. So, they have a billing cycle that sends bills more than once a month. Here's an example of a typical billing cycle for a large office.

- Patients whose last names begin with *A* to *G* are billed on the 1st of the month.

- Those with last names beginning with *H* to *N* are billed on the 8th of the month.

- Patients whose last names begin with *O* to *S* are billed on the 15th of the month.
- Those with last names beginning with *T* to *Z* are billed on the 22nd of the month.

Some offices might create their billing cycle by type of insurance. Here's an example of that type of billing cycle.

- Patients with Medicare and Medicaid are billed on the 1st of the month.
- Those with Blue Cross are billed on the 8th of the month.
- Patients with all other PPOs and HMOs are billed on the 15th of the month.
- All self-pay patients are billed on the 22nd of the month.

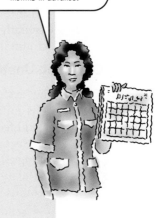

By law, your office can't change its billing cycle unless it notifies patients three months in advance.

MANAGING OVERDUE ACCOUNTS

If a patient does not pay his balance or make monthly payments as agreed, the office must collect this money. Collecting unpaid bills can be costly and time consuming for the office. A number of federal laws regulate bill collection practices. These must be followed when collecting any overdue bills.

Aging Accounts

One of your duties as an administrative medical assistant may be to track patients' accounts. You must watch them closely to make sure unpaid accounts do not become too far overdue. This process of monitoring unpaid accounts is known as "aging" the accounts.

The "age" of an account is determined by the date of the first bill, not by the date the service was provided. Here's an example.

- A patient visits the office on January 5 for a physical examination.
- The patient's first bill for the service is sent on February 1.
- The account will not become past due until the next bill is sent on March 1.

Most medical offices keep an **aging schedule** on paper or in the computer. The aging schedule contains information that's very important to the financial health of the office. Here's how the information is typically presented.

- accounts that are 30 days past due
- accounts that are 60 days past due
- accounts that are 90 days past due
- accounts that are 120 days or more past due

Generally, an account's "age" determines how you handle the account in the collection process.

Collecting Unpaid Bills

The "age" of the office's accounts also is a pretty good measure of its ability to collect its fees. In a well-run office, about 80 percent of fees should be paid within 30 days. If more than half of your fees are past due, something is probably wrong with your billing and collection procedures.

The three most common methods for collecting past due accounts are:

- sending the patient an overdue notice
- phoning to remind the patient the account is overdue
- inquiring at the patient's next office visit

Overdue Notices. This is generally the first step in the collection process. It's fairly quick and easy. You can stamp "Overdue" or "Second Notice" in red ink on the next bill sent to patients who did not pay during the 30 days after they received their first bill.

Another method is to send these patients a form letter to remind them that their account is past due. Write or type the overdue amount and any other details in the blank spaces on the form letter. If your billing is handled by computer, its software program can automatically produce either the "overdue" bill or form letter.

Whatever you send, it's a good idea to have a statement like this one printed somewhere on it:

If you recently have sent your payment, please disregard this notice. Please contact us at the phone number above if you have any questions or concerns.

This message will help prevent patients from becoming concerned or upset if they have just made their payment.

Phone Reminders. If you get no response to written overdue notices, you may have to phone the patient about his account. Always ask the patient when the office can expect to receive payment. Write the patient's response on his account card or in his computer account file. If you don't receive the payment as promised, call the patient again.

Closer Look

RULES FOR COLLECTING ACCOUNTS BY PHONE

The Fair Debt Collection Practices Act is a federal law that sets rules for collecting debts. If you call a patient about a past-due account, here are some guidelines you must follow.

- You may not call the patient at work if her employer objects to such calls.
- If you are speaking to someone else when asking for the patient or leaving a message, you cannot say the patient owes money.
- You may not call about the debt before 8:00 A.M. or after 9:00 P.M.
- You cannot contact the patient at all if he has filed for bankruptcy.
- You may not give the patient false or misleading information or make threats about further action unless the office intends to take it.
- If the patient asks in writing that such calls stop, you must do so. But you still can take legal action to collect the debt.

If you fail to follow these rules, the patient can sue the office, even if he truly owes the money.

In-Office Reminders. Only one person in the office should be responsible for reminding patients about past-due accounts. This is typically the person who works at the front desk. If this is your job, you can remind patients about overdue accounts when they come into the office for an appointment. But be sure to handle this situation privately. Give the patient a copy of the most recent overdue notice and ask when the office might expect payment.

With some computer systems, the patient's information on the screen will flash if the account is overdue. This alerts everyone who works with the patient either to discuss payment with him or refer him to someone in the office who will.

> When dealing with past-due accounts, it's a good idea to call patients the day before their appointment to remind them that their balance is due.

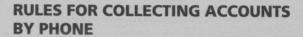

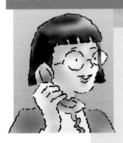

Ask the Professional

SEEING PATIENTS WITH PAST-DUE ACCOUNTS

Q: *I got a phone call from a patient who wanted to schedule a follow-up appointment with the physician. But this patient still owes us for his last three visits. Should I give him yet another appointment when he still hasn't paid for the others?*

A: It's not your job as a medical assistant to decide if a patient with a past-due balance should be seen by the physician. Schedule the appointment. Then discuss the matter privately with the physician. She may wish to continue treating this patient despite the unpaid bill. Legally, she's required to do so unless she decides to officially terminate her relationship with the patient for nonpayment of his bill. (You read about termination and termination procedures in Chapter 2.)

Collecting from a Patient's Estate. Collecting a bill for treating a patient who later died is a sensitive situation. It requires special skills and approaches. Here are some guidelines to follow.

- Don't immediately contact the patient's family about the debt. They need time to grieve and accept the death. Most offices wait until at least a week after the funeral.

- At the proper time, call the next of kin listed in the patient's chart. Offer your sympathy. Then ask for the name of the patient's executor—the person who is handling the patient's affairs after death. This will likely be a relative, a friend, or an attorney.

- Contact the executor, introduce yourself, and explain the reason for your call. Get the executor's address and send the executor the final bill.

- It's important that the bill be sent promptly. If the patient's estate doesn't have enough funds to cover the patient's debts, the court will decide the order in which the debts will be paid.

Debt-Collection Alternatives

Collecting unpaid debts is costly and time consuming to any business. Many medical offices find it easier and more effective to refer overdue accounts to collection agencies. These are companies that specialize in collecting debts. The physician or office manager must make the decision to send a patient to a collection agency.

For either a set fee or a percentage of the debt, a collection agency tries to collect the past-due amount. Its methods are much like those you would use. But its employees are professional debt collectors. They may have more success than medical office employees.

A collection agency also can sue the patient in small claims court. This is a special court that hears disputes that involve fairly small amounts of money. The largest amount that someone can be sued for varies from state to state. An advantage of small claims court is that the process is informal, and the opposing sides don't need attorneys.

A medical office can sue a patient in small claims court, too. But if it wins, it still must collect the money from the defendant. Small claims courts usually cannot force the patient to pay. So the office might still need a collection agency to collect the debt.

> Remember, if a patient's bill is turned over to a collection agency, or if the patient files for bankruptcy, you must stop trying to collect the patient's unpaid balance.

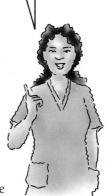

Because of all the time, trouble, and expense involved, medical offices sometimes don't seriously pursue collection of small debts from patients. If the office gives up trying to collect the money, this is called "writing off" the debt. You will learn how to make this adjustment to the patient's account later in this chapter.

The physician may wish to terminate the physician-patient relationship if the office is forced to write off the debt. The office also may report the unpaid debt to the credit bureau where it will become negative information on the patient's credit record. However, it's not your job to make these decisions.

Accounting and Bookkeeping

Accounting is an organized system for keeping track of a business's finances. One accounting activity is **bookkeeping.** This involves keeping an organized record of a business's financial activities. Accounting and bookkeeping are both very important parts of a medical office's operations.

In a large health care facility, a special department may do the accounting and billing. Other offices sometimes hire an outside firm to perform these tasks. But most offices handle the daily bookkeeping themselves. For this reason, we'll focus on bookkeeping practices in this discussion.

Bookkeeping involves keeping three kinds of financial records up to date.

- **Accounts receivable.** This is money owed to the office. This is mainly patients' accounts.
- **Accounts payable.** This is money the office owes to others. Mostly, this will be for supplies the office has purchased.
- **Petty cash.** This is a cash fund the office keeps on hand to make small purchases that may be needed quickly.

The daily financial operations of a medical office center on patients' accounts. Each day, these records change in three basic ways.

- Payments are received through the mail or electronically from patients and insurance companies.
- Patients make payments in the office by cash, check, or credit card.
- Charges for treatments and related items, such as tests and medical supplies, are added to patients' accounts.

MANUAL BOOKKEEPING SYSTEMS

The most popular systems for daily bookkeeping are the manual pegboard system and the computer system. The pegboard bookkeeping system uses a board with pegs running down the left side. The pegs hold the **day sheet** in place on the board. This form keeps a record of all patient financial activity during that day.

The day sheet is used with these other parts of the pegboard system.

- *Charge slips.* These forms are also called encounter forms or superbills. They show the services the patient received during a visit, the charges for those services, and any payment the patient made during the visit.
- *Ledger cards.* Each patient has a ledger card. It's the record of the patient's account. Charges from each visit's encounter form are recorded on it, along with payments received from the patient and the insurance company.
- *Receipts.* These forms provide a record of patients' payments made on days the office provided no new services. (If the office provided services, the patient's payment would appear on his copy of the encounter form.)

Each of these forms is printed on NCR (no carbon required) paper. The pegboard pegs and holes in the forms let you align them in the right place on top of the day sheet. Then, when you write a charge or a payment on an encounter form or a receipt, it's also recorded on the patient's ledger card and on the day sheet.

Here's all you have to do to charge a patient for services or to receive a payment on a patient's account.

1. Use the holes and pegs to place the patient's ledger card over the next empty line on the day sheet.

2. Use the holes and pegs to place the encounter form or receipt form over the next empty line on the patient's ledger card.

3. Write the charge and/or the payment in the appropriate space on the encounter form or receipt.

The amount you write will be entered automatically in the correct places on the patient's ledger card and on the day sheet. This is why the pegboard system is also called the write-it-once system. You only have to make the entry one time for it to appear on all three records.

Now let's take a closer look at each of the forms that are part of the pegboard system. Then we'll look at how to post charges, payments, and other financial information to the day sheet and to patients' accounts.

Day Sheets. The day sheet keeps track of all financial activity in patients' accounts each day. These activities include:

- charges for services to patients
- payments received from patients—in person or through the mail
- payments received from patients' health insurance plans
- adjustments to patients' accounts

> The day sheet's distribution columns provide valuable information about how your office earns its money.

You'll begin each day by putting a new day sheet on the pegboard. On busy days, you may fill the day sheet and need to use a second one. Completed day sheets are filed in date order with the most recent one on top.

The day sheet has several parts. These are the ones that involve patient accounts directly.

- *Name column.* This identifies the patient and account to which the other entries on the line apply.

- *Description column.* This describes the transaction, such as receiving a payment from a patient or an insurance company. It also could describe the services provided during an office visit. Your office will likely have standard abbreviations to be used here—such as *OV* for office visit, *I* for injection, and so on.
- *Distribution columns.* These columns are used to record charges. Each office may use them differently. In a group practice, each provider may have his own column. Other offices may assign columns to the various insurance plans they accept.
- *Payments column.* Payments received from a patient and from a patient's insurance plan are posted here.
- *Adjustments column.* An **adjustment** is an entry to change an account. These often involve reductions in fees to show insurance discounts. Other adjustments can include write-offs of uncollected fees and "bounced" checks that have been returned unpaid by a patient's bank.

The Hands On feature on page 225 gives you detailed instructions for **posting** (writing) financial entries on the day sheet.

Other parts of the day sheet aren't directly related to patient activity. But they're still important to daily bookkeeping.

- *Posting proofs section.* The day's totals are entered here and the day sheet is balanced, much like you balance a checkbook.
- *Deposit slip.* All payments are automatically recorded on this part. It's separated from the rest of the day sheet at the end of the day and included with the bank deposit of the day's payments.
- *Cash paid out section.* You'll probably make less use of this section than other parts of the day sheet. You'll read about cash paid out later in this chapter.

The day sheet is an important document because it's how the office keeps track of accounts receivable. The accounts receivable total changes each time you post a charge, payment, or adjustment to an account. You should add up the balances due on patients' ledger cards at the end of each month. This figure should equal the running total of accounts receivable that is kept on the day sheet. If it does, you know that your patient financial records are accurate.

Encounter Forms. The **encounter form** or **superbill** is the office's charge slip. It is used in both manual and computer bookkeeping systems.

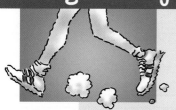

Running Smoothly

BALANCING THE DAY SHEET

What if you can't balance the day sheet?

Once you complete a day sheet, each column or section is totaled individually. Then, the posting proofs section is filled out. If the posting proofs do not balance, there's an error on the day sheet.

Here's what to do if this happens. First, take a short break. Then, return to the day sheet and follow these steps.

- Go over each transaction, one by one. Double check the entry. Be on the lookout for transposed numbers, such as an entry of 78 when you meant to write 87. This is a common error.

- For each transaction, add the fee to the previous balance or subtract the payment from the previous balance to check whether the new balance listed is correct.

- If each individual entry is correct, total each column again. Keep looking for transposed numbers.

- If you still cannot find the error, ask a colleague to check the day sheet.

- If the day sheet still doesn't balance, inform the physician or office manager.

The encounter form lists all the services, tests, and treatments the office offers, as well as the code for each one. (You'll read about these codes in Chapter 7.) You'll use this form to find the patient's charges for a visit. Here's how it will happen.

1. Write the patient's name and other personal information in the spaces provided on the form. Then, put the form with the patient's chart.

2. The physician will check off each service, test, or treatment she provides to the patient in the box next to its code and description.

3. Next, you'll use the office's fee schedule to find the fee for each checked code. You'll write each fee on the encounter form.

4. Add these fees to find the total charge for the visit and record it on the encounter form. Also record any payment received from the patient.

In a manual bookkeeping system, if you place the encounter form on the pegboard correctly, the total charge and any payment

Patient Name: _____

Patient ID #: _____ DOB: _____ Sex: _____

PCP: _____

SSN: _____ Financial Class: _____

Phone: _____ (home) _____ (work)

Medical Record #: _____ Date of Service: _____

Benefit Pkg: _____ Copay $ _____

Encounter #: _____

Service Provider: _____

Appt. Status: ☐ Scheduled ☐ Same Day ☐ Walk-in

Check-in Time: _____ Check-out Time: _____
Escorted to Exam Room: _____ Time Patient Seen: _____

Appointment Time: _____

Is Patient Being Seen in Relation to:
☐ Motor Vehicle Accident ☐ Workman's Compensation

Appointment Failure Reason:
☐ Patient Cancel ☐ No Show ☐ Walk Out ☐ PHA Cancel

TYPE OF VISIT

✓	CODE	DESCRIPTION	FEE	✓	CODE	DESCRIPTION	FEE	✓	CODE	DESCRIPTION	FEE	✓	CODE	DESCRIPTION	FEE
		OFFICE VISITS-EST.				**OFFICE VISITS-NEW CONT.**				**PREVENTATIVE, NEW**				**COUNSELING**	
	99211	Minimal			99204	Compreh.			99385	E&M 18-39			99401	15 Min.	
	99212	Focused			99205	Comp. & Complex			99386	E&M 40-64			99402	30 Min.	
	99213	Expanded				**NURSE VISIT**			99387	E&M 65 & over			99403	45 Min.	
	99214	Detailed			99211	Minimal				**CONSULTATION**			99404	60 Min.	
	99215	Compreh.				**PREVENTATIVE, EST.**			99241	Focused					
		OFFICE VISITS-NEW			99395	E&M 18-39			99242	Pre-Op Consult					
	99201	Focused			99396	E&M 40-64			99244	2nd Opinion					
	99202	Expanded			99397	E&M 65 & over									
	99203	Detailed													

PROCEDURES

✓	CODE	DESCRIPTION	FEE	✓	CODE	DESCRIPTION	FEE	✓	CODE	DESCRIPTION	FEE	✓	CODE	DESCRIPTION	FEE
	88170	Aspiration - Cyst			11200	Skin Tag Removal				**IMMUNIZATIONS/INJECTIONS**				**IMMUNIZATIONS/INJECTIONS CONT.**	
	20600	Aspiration - Joint (Small)			20550	Trigger point/Tendon Inj.			G0009	Administration Fee - Pneumovax			J2203	Triamcinolone Inj.	
	20605	Aspiration - Joint (Interm.)							G0010	Administration Fee - Hepatitis B			J3420	Vitamin B₁₂	
	20610	Aspiration - Joint (Large)				**SPECIALTY SERVICES**			95115	Allergy Injection Single				**IN-HOUSE LABORATORY**	
	16020	Burn Dressing			99070	Ace Bandage			95117	Allergy Injection Multiple			89050	Cell Count, except blood	
	69210	Ear Irrigation			E0110	Crutches			90788	Antibiotic IM			89060	Crystalanalysis	
	10120	Foreign Body Removal, Skin			29130	Finger Splint			J2910	Aurothioglucose			82948	Glucose	
	10060	I&D Abscess, simple			29125	Wrist Splint			G0008	Flu Vaccine			85013	HCT	
	90780	IV Infusion Therapy			99080	Form Completion			J1600	Gold Injection			85018	Hemoglobin Screen	
	12001	Laceration Repair, Simple				**TESTING/SCREENING**			90731	Hepatitis B			81025	Pregnancy	
	13160	Laceration Repair, Extens.			95004	Allergy - Skin Test			90741	Immune Globulin			81002	Urinalysis, Dipstick	
	64450	Medial Nerve Infiltration			92557	Audiometry			90724	Influenza			81000	Urinalysis, Full	
	17110	Molluscum/Wart Rmvl			93000	EKG			J9217	Lupron 3.75 mg			G0001	Venipuncture	
	94640	Nebulizer			92506	Hearing Screen			J9217	Lupron 7.5 mg				**OTHER PROCEDURES**	
	82270	Stool for Blood (Hemocult)			86580	PPD			J9250	Methotrexate 2-5 mg					
	12001	Suturing, Superficial			94010	Pulmonary Function			90732	Pneumovax					
	13100	Suturing, Complex			94760	Pulse Oximetry, Single			90718	Td					
	11050	Skin Les./Wart Cautery			45330	Sigmoidoscopy, Flexible			90782	Therapeutic SQ or IM					

P = PRIMARY   S = SECONDARY   S1-S9 = NUMBERED SECONDARY

DIAGNOSIS

✓	CODE	DESCRIPTION	✓	CODE	DESCRIPTION	✓	CODE	DESCRIPTION
	789.0	Abdominal Pain		780.6	Fever		462	Pharyngitis (sore throat)
	879.8	Abrasion/Laceration		704.8	Folliculitis		486	Pneumonia
	995.3	Allergic Reaction		535.5	Gastritis		V70.3	Pre-Marital Testing
	477.9	Allergic Rhinitis		558.9	Gastroenteritis		V72.81	Pre-op Cardiac Exam
	285.9	Anemia		274.9	Gout		V72.83	Pre-op Exam, Other
	413.9	Angina		V72.3	Gyn Exam		601.0	Prostatits
	300.00	Anxiety		784.0	Headache		600	Prostatism
	716.90	Arthritis		389.9	Hearing Loss		782.1	Rash
	427.9	Arrhythmia		536.8	Heartburn/Indigestion		569.3	Rectal Bleeding
	493.90	Asthma		573.3	Hepatitis		530.81	Reflux
	611.72	Breast Lump		455.6	Hemorrhoids		V81.2	Screening for Cardiac Condition
	490	Bronchitis		553.9	Hernia		780.3	Seizure Disorder
	727.3	Bursitis		401.9	Hypertension (NOS)		473.9	Sinusitis
	354.0	Carpal Tunnel Syndrome		272.4	Hyperlipidemia		848.9	Strain/Sprain
	682.9	Cellulitis		242.00	Hyperthyroidism		438	Stroke
	786.50	Chest Pain		251.2	Hypoglycemia		305.90	Substance Abuse
	575.1	Cholecystitis		380.4	Impacted Cerumen		099.9	STD
	372.3	Conjunctivitis		780.52	Insomnia		727.00	Tenosynovitis, Tendonitis
	496	COPD		564.1	Irritable Bowel Syndrome		451.9	Thrombophlebitis
	414.9	Coronary Artery Disease		719.40	Joint Pain		246.9	Thyroid Disease
	290.9	Dementia		592.0	Kidney Stones		435.9	TIA
	311	Depression		464.0	Laryngitis		463	Tonsillitis
	692.9	Dermatitis		724.2	Low Back Pain		011.90	Tuberculosis
	250.01	Diabetes, IDDM		710.0	Lupus		465.9	Upper Respiratory Infection
	250.00	Diabetes, NIDDM		V70.0	Medical Exam/Physical		599.0	Urinary Tract Infection
	558.9	Diarrhea		346.9	Migraine		V04.8	Vaccination, Flu
	562.10	Diverticular Disease		278.0	Obesity		V03.9	Vaccination, Pneumovax
	780.4	Dizziness		382.9	Otitis Media		616.10	Vaginitis
	995.2	Drug Reaction		614.9	Pelvic Inflammatory Disease		424.9	Valvular Heart Disease
	782.3	Edema		533.9	Peptic Ulcer Disease		079.9	Viral Syndrome
	780.7	Fatigue/Tiredness/Malaise		443.9	Peripheral Vascular Disease			

Comments: _____

PREVIOUS BALANCE	$
TODAY'S CHARGES	$
PAYMENT	$
BALANCE	$

RETURN APPOINTMENT:
_____ Days _____ Weeks _____ Months
APPT. LENGTH: _____ PROVIDER: _____

APPT. REASON: _____

PROVIDER SIGNATURE: _____

Adult

Philadelphia
Health Associates
Tax ID #23-2350500
PHA Group # PH75923

☐ 3550 Market Street
Philadelphia, PA 19104
(215) 823-8660

☐ The Bourse Building
111 S. Independence Mall
East • 7th Floor
Philadelphia, PA 19106
(215) 625-9100

PHA-019 (6/95)

OTHER DIAGNOSIS

✓	CODE	DESCRIPTION	✓	CODE	DESCRIPTION

Here's an example of a standard encounter form and charge slip.

DATE	FAMILY MEMBER	PROFESSIONAL SERVICE		CHARGE	CREDITS		NEW BALANCE	PREVIOUS BALANCE	NAME
					PAYMENTS	ADJ			

You **PAID** this amount

This is a **STATEMENT** of your account to date

DIAGNOSIS OR NATURE OF ILLNESS OR INJURY:

REF No.	ICD-9 CODE	DESCRIPTION
1.	( )	
2.	( )	
3.	( )	
4.	( )	

Correlate diagnosis to procedure by using the reference numbers listed above

CPT	PROCEDURE	ICD-9 Ref. No.	FEE
	Office Visit - New Patient		
☐ 99201	Focused		$
☐ 99202	Expanded		$
☐ 99203	Detailed		$
☐ 99204	Comprehensive		$
☐ 99205	Comprehensive		$
	Office Visit - Established Patient		
☐ 99211	Minimal		$
☐ 99212	Focused		$
☐ 99213	Expanded		$
☐ 99214	Detailed		$
☐ 99215	Comprehensive		$
	Office Consultation		
☐ 99241	Focused		$
☐ 99242	Expanded		$
☐ 99243	Detailed		$
☐ 99244	Comprehensive		$
☐ 99245	Comprehensive		$
☐			$
☐			$
☐			$
☐			$
☐			$
☐			$

CPT	PROCEDURE	ICD-9 Ref. No.	FEE
	General Services		
☐ 95115	Allergen Immunotherapy, Single Injection		
☐ 69210	Removal Impacted Cerumen		$
☐ 45330	Sigmoidoscopy, Flexible Fiberoptic		$
☐ 93015	Cardiovascular Stress Test		$
☐ 94010	Spirometry		$
☐ 94060	Spirometry with BD		$
☐ 93000	ECG, with Interp. and Report		$
☐ 99000	Handling and/or Conveyance Specimen		$
☐ 86580	Tuberculosis, Intradermal		$
	Laboratory		
☐ 36415*	Routine Venipuncture		
☐ 86255	Fluorescent Antibody, Screen		$
☐ 85032	Hemogram (CBC)		$
	Manual Differential		$
☐ 80050	General Health Screen Panel		$
☐ 80162	Digoxin, RIA		$
☐ 82948	Glucose; Blood		$
☐ 82270	Blood; Occult, Feces, Screen.		$
☐ 85014	Hematocrit		$
☐ 86308	Heterophile Antibodies (Monotype)		$
☐ 85049	Platelet Count		$
☐ 84132	Potassium; Blood		$
☐ 85610	Prothrombin Time		$
☐ 80194	Quinidine, Blood		$
☐ 86592	Syphilis Test, Qualitative		$
☐ 81000	Urinalysis, by Reagent Strip		$
☐			$
☐			$
☐			$
☐			$

CPT	PROCEDURE	ICD-9 Ref. No.	FEE
	Immunization Injections		
☐ 90702	Diphtheria and Tetanus Toxoids		$
☐ 90656	Influenza Virus Vaccine		$
☐ 90732	Pneumococcal Vaccine, Polyvalent		$
☐ 36000	Therapeutic Injection Specify Material:		$
☐ 90765	Therapeutic IV Specify Material:		$
☐ J3420	Inj. B-12		$
☐ J0290	Inj. Ampicillin, 500 mg.		$

DATE OF SERVICE _____

PLACE OF SERVICE:
☐ Office   ☐ Inpatient hospital
☐ Skilled nursing facility   ☐ Nursing Home

REFERRING MD: _____

SIGNATURE OF PHYSICIAN _____   Date _____

WILLIAM PARKER, P.C.
125 GREEN STREET
BURTON, OH 45123

TAX I.D. # 123456
S.S. NO. 000-00-0000
UPIN #E00000

1070

FORM 159993 ITEM 7302 COLWELL SYSTEMS 1.800.637.1140

Here's an example of an encounter form that would be used with the pegboard system.

you write on it also will appear on the patient's account ledger card and on the day sheet.

Some encounter forms are three-part forms.

- Keep the top, original form for the office's records.
- Submit the middle copy to the patient's insurance company.
- Give the bottom copy to the patient. It's a record of services and charges as well as a receipt for any payment made that day.

Ledger Cards. The ledger card is the financial record for a patient. The top part of the card contains the patient's personal and insurance information. The bottom part lists the charges, payments, and adjustments made to the patient's account.

Some practices use photocopies of patients' ledger cards as bills. They copy the cards that show balances due and mail the copies to the patients. If your office follows this practice, make sure nothing other than the name and address of the person being billed is visible in the window of the envelope. If any other information on the bill shows, it is a violation of the patient's privacy.

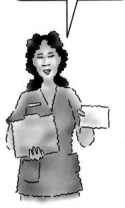

You should keep a patient's ledger card as long as you keep his medical record. Both are legal documents.

Posting Charges and Payments

Whether your office uses copies of ledger cards as bills or sends out bills prepared by the computer, the information on them should be the same. Both should show not only the total charge, but also the specific services provided during the visit. Most computer-produced bills will show the charge for each service as well.

Only the total charge for the visit is recorded on the day sheet, however. The Hands On procedure on page 226 gives you specific guidance on posting charges to the patient's account.

The payments the office receives may include:

- insurance payments
- patient checks or money orders received in the mail
- patient payments made in person with credit cards, debit cards, checks, or cash

Procedures for posting these payments are outlined in the Hands On procedure on page 227.

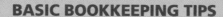

Closer Look — BASIC BOOKKEEPING TIPS

Here are some practices that will help you keep patient financial records in good order.

- Always use ink (black ink is best) when making entries. Don't use pencil.

- Check your math before writing the financial information across the top of the encounter form and onto the patient ledger and day sheet.

- Write neatly. Be especially careful to form your numbers clearly.

- If you make a mistake, draw a single line through the incorrect entry, record the correct information, and initial the change. Never use white-out or erase or scribble through errors

- If necessary, reenter the correct transaction on a new line on the ledger and day sheet.

- When an entry is complete, double check it for accuracy.

Overpayments and Refunds

Overpayment of an account is more common than you might think. It can happen easily when you are collecting some money from the patient as well as billing one or more insurance companies for the patient's charges.

Sometimes, payments from the patient and his insurance may total more than the charge for the visit. This will show on the patient's ledger card as a **credit balance.** A credit balance is different from a balance due. A balance due is what is owed on the account. A credit balance is an overpayment.

You show a credit balance by placing brackets around the amount in the balance-due column—for example, [$125.64]. Brackets are used in accounting to show the opposite of a column's normal meaning. In this case, it means that the amount in the balance due column is not what the patient owes, but what the office owes the patient or insurance company instead.

The office is legally and ethically required to return insurance overpayments to the insurance company. Overpayments by a patient are handled in one of two ways.

- The patient's payment stays on the account as a credit to be applied to future charges.

- The office mails the patient a check for the amount of the overpayment.

How patients' overpayments are handled depends on office policy and on the size of the overpayment. In many offices, overpayments of less than $5 are left on the account as a credit balance. Overpayments of $5 or more are refunded. The Hands On procedure on page 228 will guide you in processing credit balances and issuing refunds.

Credit Adjustments

The adjustments column on the ledger card and day sheet is used to make adjustments to the patient's account that don't involve charges or payments. There are two basic types of adjustments—credit adjustments and debit adjustments.

The most common reason for making a credit adjustment to an account involves insurance. Most medical offices are providers for one or more insurance plans. This means they've agreed to accept lower fees set by the insurance company instead of the office's normal fees.

> Accounting is easier to understand if you remember that a _debit_ is an addition to what is owed, and a _credit_ is a reduction to what is owed.

You must charge every patient the same fee for the same service. That's the fee for the service that is shown on the office's fee schedule. But when the insurance payment is received, it will be for the agreed-on fee. This will be less than the fee you charged to the account.

You'll post the insurance payment in the payments column of the day sheet and ledger card. But then you must write off the difference between the payment and the fee-schedule fee that you charged. You do this by making a credit adjustment for the difference in the adjustments column of the day sheet and ledger card.

Suppose, for example, your office charges $40 for an office visit. But the agreed-on fee with the patient's insurance plan is only $35. You would post $40 in the charges column. Then, when the insurance payment is received, you would enter $35 in the payment column and $5 in the adjustments column to arrive at the agreed-on amount for this service.

Here are two more examples of credit adjustments.

- The physician gives a nurse a 25% professional discount on an office visit. You would enter the $40 fee from the fee schedule in the charges column. In the description column, you would indicate an office visit with a 25% professional discount. Then you would make a $10 (25% of $40) credit adjustment in the adjustments column. This would leave the nurse with a balance due of $30 for this visit.

- A patient owes the office $1,200. You haven't been able to collect it, so the account is turned over to a collection agency. In most offices, you will write off this balance to keep better control over accounts receivable. So you would show "collection agency" in the description column and put $1,200 in the adjustments column. This would bring the patient's balance to 0.

The Hands On procedure on page 229 provides guidance for posting credit adjustments.

Debit Adjustments

Credit adjustments generally reduce a patient's account balance. Debit adjustments add to or increase the patient's balance.

Let's go back to the last example of a credit adjustment. Suppose the collection agency collects the $1,200 from the patient and sends in a check for that amount. Remember that the patient's balance has been adjusted to 0. You must charge money to the account in order to post the collection agency's payment. Otherwise, the account will have a credit balance of $1,200.

Since these are not new charges, you would not add the $1,200 in the charges column. Instead, you will make a $1,200 debit adjustment in the adjustments column. Then, when you post the collection agency's check, the patient's balance will be 0 again.

The Hands On procedure on page 229 provides instructions for posting collection agency payments. Here are two other examples of when you will need to make a debit adjustment to a patient's account.

- You've already read that insurance overpayments must be refunded to the insurance company. To eliminate the overpayment, you must debit the account. Write the amount of the refund in brackets in the adjustments column. In the description column, write *refund to insurance carrier*. The Hands On procedure on page 228 contains guidelines for making such refunds.

- A patient's check is returned by the bank marked NSF. This stands for *not sufficient funds*. It means the patient doesn't have enough money in his account for the bank to pay the check. Because the check was no good, you have to put the charges back on the account because the patient still owes them. Most offices also charge the patient a fee for returned checks. The Hands On procedure on page 230 gives you instructions about how to handle this.

Cash Paid Out. From time to time, the physician may take cash from the payments you receive. If this happens, your bank deposit for that day is going to be short by the amount taken out. The best way to handle this is to write the amount taken in the cash paid out section of the day sheet. Have the physician sign on the description line for the entry.

The cash paid out section has another use too. Sometimes, when insurance companies overpay, they don't expect refunds. Instead, they apply the overpayment to what they owe on another patient's bill. When you get the insurance check for that other patient, it will be short by the amount of the previous overpayment.

When this happens, post the full amount expected from the insurance company in the payments section. Then, use the cash paid out section to account for the difference. You do that by writing the amount of the shortage in the cash paid out section and noting *insurance refund applied to account of* [*the other patient's name*] on the description line.

COMPUTER ACCOUNTING SYSTEMS

Most medical office accounting software is easy to use. Computer bookkeeping programs perform most of the functions of the pegboard system. But they do so much faster. Instead of writing entries, you key them into the computer. Plus, you never have to worry about being unable to read the handwriting on the day sheet.

Besides these advantages, computer systems offer several others.

- They do all the math—such as adding up fees, calculating adjustments, and balancing each day's totals—without error.

- They can print out bills and receipts for patients and insurance companies. Many systems also can write refund checks.

- Some programs can manage electronic banking between the office and the bank.

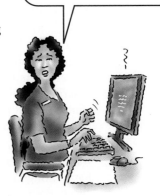

If you use a computer bookkeeping program, make sure it has a good backup system. That way, if the computer crashes, your entries won't be lost.

Posting to Computer Accounts

If you understand the manual bookkeeping system, you'll have no trouble using a computer-based program. The software will take you though each process. For example, to post a payment to a patient's account, here's all you have to do.

- Bring up the patient's account from the accounts database.
- Key in the source and amount of the payment, the allowed amount for the service, and any needed adjustments.

The computer will perform all the calculations automatically and without error. In addition, several of the Hands On procedures at the end of this chapter provide steps for performing the task using a computer system as well as a manual one.

Computer Accounting Reports

Computer bookkeeping systems keep track of the individual patient postings you make during the day. At the end of the day, they produce a daily report that you can print out. This report looks much like a day sheet and contains the same basic information.

Other daily and weekly reports provide the same information found at the bottom of the day sheet in a manual system. At any time, you can ask the computer for a report on the office's year-to-date (or for any period of time you wish) financial summary. Some programs also can create reports on the income produced by each physician in a group practice.

Banking Matters

Several things are important in choosing a bank for the office's business account.

- *The bank's location.* Because you probably will be making a deposit at the end of each day, a nearby bank would be the most convenient.
- *Monthly service fees.* Most banks charge the office each month to have an account there. Some banks, however, don't charge any monthly fee if the account's balance doesn't fall below a stated level.
- *Returned check fees.* Some banks charge a fee if a check you deposit in your account is returned unpaid because the writer did not have enough money in her account to pay it.
- *Overdraft protection.* This service guarantees that the bank will pay the checks you write even if not enough money is

in the office's account. The bank usually charges a fee for this protection from "bouncing" a check.

- *Special services.* Many banks offer special programs to attract small businesses such as medical offices to bank there. For example, the bank might pay the office interest on the money in its checking account.

MAKING DEPOSITS

The first thing you should do when a check comes into the office is check to be sure it is made out to your office and filled in correctly. Next, you must endorse the check. This involves writing the name of the physician or medical office and account number on the back of the check. The office should have a stamp with this information already on it. All you have to do is stamp the back of the check in the place marked for endorsement. If the office doesn't have an endorsement stamp, you should get one.

When the day's payments have been received, posted, and processed, add all the checks, credit card receipts, and cash received. The total should match the total of the payments column on the day sheet. If it does, you're ready to prepare the day's receipts for deposit in the office's bank account. The Hands On procedure on page 231 gives you step-by-step instructions for doing this.

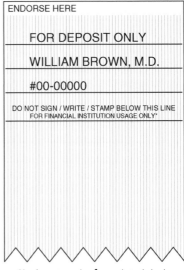

Here's an example of an endorsed check.

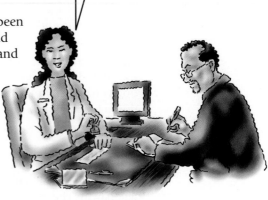

Endorse checks as soon as you receive them. That way, if they're lost or stolen, no one else can cash them.

Closer Look — MORE ABOUT CHECKS

Certain kinds of checks are more "secure" than the personal checks patients may write to pay on their accounts.

- Certified checks are written from the patient's account and stamped by the bank. The bank guarantees that it's holding enough money in the patient's account to pay the check.

- Cashier's checks are written by the bank and sold to the customer for the amount of the check plus an additional fee. This process gives the receiver of the check confidence that it's good.

- Money orders aren't true checks, but they do guarantee payment just like cashier's checks. Banks, the U.S. Postal Service, and some stores and businesses sell these to customers.

The deposit can be mailed to the bank or dropped in the bank's secure night deposit box. But if the deposit includes any cash, you should take it directly to a bank teller. Always get a receipt from the teller for any deposits that contain cash.

WRITING CHECKS

Another of your administrative duties may be handling accounts payable—that is, paying the office's bills. Accounts payable usually include such things as:

- rent and utilities
- refunds to patients and insurance companies
- payment for supplies and services
- repayment to the office's petty cash fund
- employees' salaries
- taxes

Accounts payable usually are paid by check. You may produce these checks on the computer or write them by hand. In either case, you probably won't be signing the checks. In most offices, the office manager, business manager, or physician signs the accounts payable checks. Some offices require two signatures on checks, especially if they're over a certain amount.

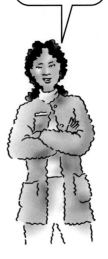

Your office's bank has signature cards that determine who can sign accounts payable checks.

Here are some points to remember when you prepare accounts payable checks.

- Be sure you make the check payable to the correct name of the person or business.
- Place the current date on the check.
- Enter the payment amount in both words and numbers.
- Put the reason for the check on its memo line for reference.
- Record the date, check number, amount of the check, and who it's payable to in the checking account register.
- Subtract the check's amount from the register balance.
- Post the payment to the appropriate category or account in the office's financial records.

If you are preparing checks by hand, be sure your handwriting is clear.

In addition to the checkbook register, the office should keep a log book of all checks written. Along with the date, number, and amount of the check, the log should include why the check was written—for example, office supplies, payroll taxes, monthly credit card bill, and so on.

DEALING WITH BANK STATEMENTS

Banks mail a monthly statement to account holders. This statement shows all account activity since the previous statement. It lists the following information:

- all checks written and their amounts
- all deposits made and their amounts
- all electronic transactions
- any service charges

You must reconcile each monthly statement. This means you must compare it with your office records for the account. The main office record you'll use is the checkbook register. Here's what to do.

1. Compare the amounts of all checks and deposits listed on the statement with their listing in the register. Verify that the information is identical.
2. Make a check mark in the register for each check the statement shows has been paid by the bank.
3. Make a check mark in the register for each deposit the statement shows was received by the bank.

4. Total all deposits that have no check marks in the register. Add that total to the ending balance shown on the statement. This is the revised ending balance.

5. Total all the checks that have no check marks in the register. Subtract that total from the revised ending balance you calculated in step 4.

6. Subtract from the register balance any fees and charges shown on the statement that are not recorded in the register. (Enter these fees and charges in the register so the register is balanced.)

7. The balance you reach in step 6 should equal the balance you reached in step 5. If it does not, there is a problem. Check your math and make sure the numbers are all correct. If no errors in the math are found, there could be a problem with your checking account.

Ordering Supplies

Like all businesses, one of your office's goals is financial success. You've already read how billing, collections, and bookkeeping practices contribute to this goal. Keeping the office's expenses down does too.

There are many ways to save money when buying office supplies. Here are just a few of them.

- A purchasing cooperative (co-op) allows the office to join with others in buying supplies. The co-op's members benefit from the lower prices that go with large orders.

- Some suppliers offer price discounts for prompt payment.

- Large warehouse-type sellers and companies with discount catalogs also offer low prices.

When buying supplies, compare the items' current prices to those on old invoices in your files.

Finding the best deals can take time. But the savings can be worth the effort, especially for items you use a lot.

There are things other than cost to consider in deciding what and where to buy. Consider the following:

- All supplies should be high quality, not just inexpensive. Many offices use several suppliers to get this mix of good quality and good price.

- Office supply companies often deliver for free. Office warehouse chains may charge a delivery fee or require a minimum order for free delivery.

RECEIVING AND PAYING FOR SUPPLIES

Arriving supplies should always have a **packing slip** with them that lists the items the delivery contains. Always compare the packing slip to the shipment's actual contents. This is a check to make sure the order is accurate and complete.

If all the goods were received, initial the slip. Place all packing slips in a bills-pending file so they can be compared to the **invoice,** or bill, when it arrives. If the supplies were paid for in advance, place the packing slip in the appropriate accounts-paid file. If any items were missing, mark them on the packing slip. Then, contact the company.

Invoices for supplies and other bills the office has not yet paid should be kept in a bills-pending file. This will help prevent them from being lost or misplaced. Bills may be paid daily, weekly, every two weeks, or monthly. Generally, office policy will determine how often accounts payable checks are written.

Petty Cash

Most offices keep a petty cash fund to make small purchases. For example, suppose you run out of file folders and need more right away. Since it will take time to get more from your office supplier, you could buy a box at a local store to use until the new supply arrives. You would take money from petty cash to pay for this small purchase.

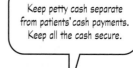

Keep petty cash separate from patients' cash payments. Keep all the cash secure.

The value of a petty cash always remains the same. This means that when you take money out, you replace it with the receipt for money spent. The cash remaining in the fund and the total of the receipts should always equal the set value of the fund.

The petty cash fund usually is renewed once a month. This is done by writing and cashing an accounts payable check for an amount that equals the total of the receipts in the fund. The receipts are removed and filed, and the money from the cashed check is put in the fund.

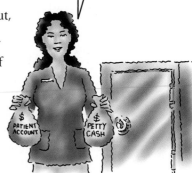

Payroll

Many medical offices hire an outside service to keep its payroll records and issue the paychecks for its staff. But in some offices, these checks will be written by an administrative medical assistant.

Generally, paychecks will be written and issued on one of the following schedules:

- weekly (52 pay periods per year)
- biweekly (26 pay periods per year)
- monthly (12 pay periods per year)

Your employer decides the pay period in your office. Usually, all the employees are paid on the same schedule.

DEDUCTIONS AND WITHHOLDINGS

Writing payroll checks requires more than just knowing each employee's pay rate. A number of amounts must be deducted from employees' pay. Here are the common payroll deductions.

- health, life, or disability insurance premiums
- employee contributions to the company-sponsored retirement plan
- court-ordered withholdings to pay a debt the employee owes
- federal taxes

In most states, state income tax must be withheld, too. Many cities and towns also tax the earnings of people who live or work there.

Federal Taxes

The federal taxes you must withhold from employees' paychecks are:

- federal income tax (FIT)
- Social Security (also known as FICA)
- Medicare

All three of these withholdings are based on the amount of the employee's earnings. In general, the greater the employee's pay, the larger the amount that is withheld. In 2005, you would have withheld 6.2% of the employee's pay for Social Security and 1.45% for Medicare.

The size of the FIT withholding is affected by the employee's marital status and by the number of exemptions the employee claims. This information is contained on the employee's W-4 form. If an employee has no W-4 form on file, you must withhold FIT from her paycheck at the highest rate. That is the tax rate for a single person with no dependents.

The W-4 Form. Each employee must complete a federal W-4 form on the first day of hire. The W-4 form contains the employee's name, address, Social Security number, marital status,

Closer Look   EMPLOYEE RECORDS

No matter who does your office payroll, the office should have a personnel file on each employee. The file should contain the following items and information:

- employee's original job application or résumé
- job references
- salary or hourly rate at time of hire
- dates and amounts of pay raises
- performance reviews and evaluations
- all employee withholding authorization forms, such as W-4 forms
- pension plan, health, and life insurance paperwork
- vital facts such as employee's date of birth, name of spouse, address and phone number, and name and daytime phone number of an emergency contact person

and number of exemptions she claims. In general, employees can claim one exemption for each person who depends on their income. An employee's dependents usually are her spouse or minor children.

Calculating Federal Withholdings

You can find out easily how much federal taxes to withhold from each employee's check by using tax tables provided by the U.S. Internal Revenue Service (IRS). Combined tax tables found in IRS publications for businesses calculate the withholding for FIT, Social Security, and Medicare for you.

The tables tell how much to withhold for weekly, biweekly, monthly, and other payroll periods. Your office's payroll period and the marital status of the employee will determine which table to use. If an employee's wages are greater than the highest bracket on the table, you will have to use one of the other methods described in the publication to calculate the withholding.

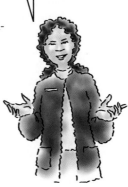

Employees who earn more than $90,000 pay Social Security and Medicare taxes only on the first $90,000. You stop withholding these taxes when their income for the year reaches that amount.

TAXES PAID BY THE EMPLOYER

An employer must match the amount withheld from each employee's check for Social Security and Medicare. Suppose, for example, that you withhold $150 from an employee's check for these taxes. The office must pay $300 to the IRS—$150 for the employee's withholding and $150 for the employer's match.

Each pay period, or at least once a month, you will write an accounts payable check to the IRS for the federal taxes you have withheld from employees' paychecks. This check will be for the total of the following amounts:

- all the federal income tax withheld from employees' pay

- all the Medicare tax withheld from employees' pay plus the employer's matching contribution.

- all the Social Security tax withheld plus the employer's matching contribution

The medical office's accountant will give you the federal deposit forms you will need to include with the check.

The office's accountant will calculate how much federal unemployment tax (FUTA) your employer must pay. This tax is paid either quarterly (every three months) or once a year. Most states also require employers to pay a state unemployment tax. The accountant also will calculate how much this state tax will be.

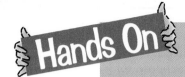

PREPARING AND SENDING A BILL

6-1

It's important that charges for services are billed and collected regularly. Follow these procedures in sending patients a statement of their account.

1. Prepare statements according to the monthly billing cycle followed by the office. Some offices do all billing at the same time each month. Others divide the alphabet and send bills two or more times per month, depending on the patient's last name.

2. Gather patient ledgers for accounts that show outstanding balances. Send statements only to patients who have a balance due on their account.

3. Photocopy the ledger card or prepare a printed statement. Make sure each bill shows the following information:
   - patient's name
   - name and address of person responsible for payment
   - date of visit, an itemized list of services provided, and the charge for each service
   - any unpaid balance carried over from the previous month
   - any insurance payments, patient co-pays, or other patient payments received since the last bill
   - the total amount that remains due

4. Identify and mark bills showing balances that are past due.

5. Discuss with the physician or office manager any further action to be taken on the past-due accounts. Follow through on his instructions for collecting these accounts.

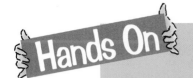

POSTING ENTRIES ON A DAY SHEET

6-2

The day sheet is the central record of patient financial activity in a manual pegboard system. Even if you use a computerized financial program, it's important to understand the day sheet and pegboard system. This is the process on which computer systems are based.

1. Align the new day sheet and blank charge slips on the pegboard.

2. Fill in the date and page number.

3. Carefully copy all balances and totals forwarded from the previous day's sheet into the correct boxes on the new day sheet.

4. Arrange patients' ledger cards in order of patient appointment times for the day.

5. When a patient arrives, pull her ledger card and attach a charge slip/encounter form (superbill) to her chart.

6. At the end of the patient's visit, put her ledger card on the pegboard, aligning it with her name on the day sheet.

7. Place the patient's charge slip/encounter form (superbill) over her ledger on the pegboard, aligning the first blank line on the ledger with the entry strip on the charge slip.

8. Write the date, patient's name, name of the insured, and any previous balance on the charge slip in the correct space.

9. Enter the total charge and any payment received in the correct columns on the charge slip.

10. Determine the final balance by adding any previous balance to that day's charge and subtracting any payments. Enter the final balance on the ledger/day sheet.

11. When the posting is complete, give the bottom copy of the charge slip to the patient. This will serve as her record of the visit and her receipt for any payment.

Hands On

POSTING CHARGES TO A PATIENT'S ACCOUNT

6-3

Careful documentation of services provided and fees owed is important to the smooth running of a medical office. Follow these guidelines to post charges to a patient's account.

1. Take the charge slip from the patient.
   - Check that the charge slip is complete and signed by the physician or other service provider.
   - Make sure the name on the charge slip matches the name on the patient ledger card or patient account on the computer.

2. If using a ledger card, post the total amount of the visit's charges in the charge column of the card. List each service in the description column.
   - Use abbreviations such as *OV* for office visit, *PE* for physical examination, *I* for injection, *LAB* for laboratory services, etc.
   - Provide a key to the abbreviations used at the bottom of the ledger card.

3. If using a computer, post each service separately on the charge screen.
   - Most programs require you to enter a code for each service.
   - When you enter the code, the computer will post the proper charge for the service automatically.

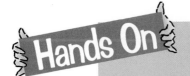

POSTING PAYMENTS TO A PATIENT'S ACCOUNT

6-4

As with all other bookkeeping procedures, accuracy in recording payments received is important for an office's financial records to remain in order. Follow these steps to post a payment to a patient's account.

1. Align the patient's ledger card on the day sheet. If the patient is paying for services received on this visit, the charge slip should also be in place on the pegboard.

2. Enter the patient's name and previous balance in the proper columns. If using a charge slip, enter its number in the receipt number column.

3. Enter the posting date in the date column.

4. Enter the type of payment—personal check (pers. ck.), insurance check (ins. ck.), credit card (MC, VISA), etc.—in the description column.

5. Enter the amount of payment in the payment column and in the deposit section of the day sheet in the cash or checks column.

6. Subtract the payment amount from the previous balance and record the new balance.
   - If only a payment is being made, there will be no entry in the fee area.
   - If you made an entry in the fee area, find the new balance. To do this, add the new charge to the previous balance before subtracting the payment.

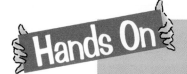

PROCESSING CREDIT BALANCES AND ISSUING REFUNDS

6-5

Occasionally, a patient's payment and his insurance company's payment will total more than the patient owes. When this happens, a credit balance will exist on the account. Follow these steps to handle this situation.

1. Pull the ledger cards of patients with credit balances. Do this at least monthly, or more often if called for by office procedures.

2. Place the ledger card on the pegboard, taking care to align it correctly.

3. Enter the insurance payment for the patient in the payments column.

4. Determine the amount by which the charges must be adjusted and enter it in the adjustment column.
   - This amount will be the difference between the insurance company's fee schedule and the office's full fee for each service billed.
   - Remember that many insurance companies require the office to accept what they pay as payment in full.

5. Subtract the adjustment amount and insurance payment from the previous balance to arrive at the balance due.
   - If the adjustment and insurance payment total more than the previous balance, the balance due will be less than zero.
   - A balance due of less than zero means that a surplus of funds, called a "credit balance," exists in the account.
   - A credit balance is posted [in brackets] in the balance column to show that it is money due the patient (or insurance company) and not owed to the office.

6. Return the account balance to zero by refunding the amount of the credit balance.

7. Write the amount of the refund [in brackets] in the adjustments column to show that it is a debit adjustment, and not a credit.

8. Write a check for the refund amount to whomever the credit balance is owed—the patient or the insurance company.

9. Document the refund in the description column of a patient's ledger card and in the office's check register.

10. Mail the refund check.

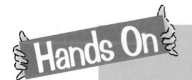

POSTING A CREDIT ADJUSTMENT

6-6

For a number of reasons, medical offices generally do not collect the full amount they charge. When the amount collected is less than the charge, an adjustment must be made to balance the account. Follow these steps to make a credit adjustment.

1. Align the patient's ledger card on the day sheet.

2. Record the date, the patient's name, and his previous account balance in the proper columns.

3. Record the amount of the adjustment in the adjustment column.

4. Record the reason for the adjustment in the description column—for example, professional discount, insurance adjustment, write-off, etc.

5. Subtract the amount of the adjustment from the previous balance and record the new balance in the balance column.

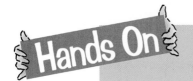

POSTING COLLECTION AGENCY PAYMENTS

6-7

Follow these steps to accept payment by a collection agency of charges collected on a long overdue account.

1. Pull the patient's ledger card and align it directly on the day sheet. No charge slip or receipt is needed.

2. Enter the patient's previous balance on the day sheet. (If the account was zeroed when it was turned over for collection, the patient's old balance due should be debited back in on her ledger card.)

3. Post the date, amount received, and the description "Received on Account" (or ROA) on the ledger card.

4. Do a credit adjustment to zero out any balance remaining. This will represent any uncollected amount plus the collection agency's fee.

Hands On   POSTING NSF CHECKS   6-8

Occasionally, a bank will return a patient's check to the office for NSF, or "not sufficient funds." Because the patient didn't have enough money in his account to pay the check, the amount of the check must be added back into the patient's account. Follow these steps to do this type of debit adjustment.

1. Pull the patient's ledger card and align it with the first available line on the current day sheet.

2. Write the amount of the check in the payment column [in brackets] to indicate that it is a debit adjustment, not a credit to the account.

3. Write "Check returned for NSF" in the description column.

4. If your bank charges a fee for returned checks, write the amount of this fee in the charges column.

5. Write "Bank fee for returned check" in the description column.

6. Add these two amounts to the patient's previous balance to determine her new account balance.

7. Follow office policy for notifying the patient of the returned check and adjustment.

8. Remember to subtract the amount of the returned check and the bank fee from the office's checking account balance.

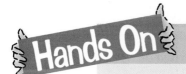 **PREPARING A BANK DEPOSIT**   **6-9**

Follow these procedures to prepare the payments received in the office for deposit in the office's bank account.

1. Separate checks and cash. Make sure the office's endorsement stamp is on the back of each check.

2. Organize cash in order of the size of bills.
   - Group all $1s, $5s, $10s, $20s, etc., together and facing in the same direction.
   - Some banks also require that coins be grouped and wrapped.

3. Count the cash and record the total amount on the deposit slip.

4. List each check separately on the deposit slip.
   - Place the patient's name in the left column and the amount of the check in the right column.
   - Make a copy of the deposit slip for the office record.

5. Total the amount of cash and checks and enter it on the deposit slip. This total should equal the total in the payments column of the day sheet.

6. Place the cash, checks, and deposit slip in an envelope to take to the bank.

7. Enter the date and amount of the deposit in the office's checkbook register.

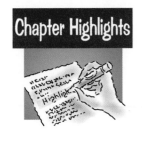

Chapter Highlights

- The financial health of a medical office is based on its ability to collect the fees it charges.

- Credit arrangements, monthly billing, and attention to the collection of aging accounts help keep office finances running smoothly and efficiently.

- As an administrative medical assistant, you may be responsible for posting charges, payments, and adjustments to patients' accounts.

- You also may be responsible for making bank deposits, keeping records of accounts payable, and even doing the office payroll.

- To carry out your bookkeeping responsibilities effectively, you must record all transactions promptly and accurately.

- Computers have made office bookkeeping much easier, but to use computer systems properly, you must understand the accounting principles of the older manual systems.

Chapter 7

MEDICAL CODING

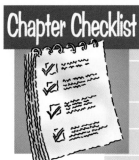

Chapter Checklist

- Explain what coding is and why it is used
- Describe the relationship between diagnostic coding, procedural coding, and reimbursement
- Describe how the ICD-9-CM is organized
- List the steps in identifying a proper diagnostic code
- Name the common errors in diagnostic coding
- Perform diagnostic coding
- Describe how the CPT-4 is organized and used
- Summarize the factors that determine which E/M code to assign a patient visit
- Understand HCPCS codes and surgical packages
- Perform procedural coding
- Explain how ICD and CPT codes and coding methods are similar

In the simplest terms, medical coding is assigning a number to a verbal statement or description. But in practice, this process is anything but simple. It's a complex task that requires accuracy, medical knowledge, and careful attention to detail.

Coding is also one of the most important jobs you may be asked to do as an administrative medical assistant. The codes you use to describe a patient's diagnosis and treatment will determine what the patient's health insurance plan will pay.

If the codes you assign are incorrect or incomplete, payment may be reduced, delayed, or denied. Since most of a medical office's income generally comes from insurance, this makes coding a critical task.

Coded Messages

Medical coding replaces verbal descriptions of diseases, injuries, conditions, and services with numeric, or number, codes. There are two types of codes.

- *Diagnostic codes.* There's a code for nearly every illness, injury, or condition a patient may have. These codes come from the *International Classification of Diseases, Ninth Revision, Clinical Modification.* Medical professionals call this book the ICD-9-CM. This book is updated annually, so your office should purchase a new copy each year.

- *Procedure codes.* The source of these codes is the fourth edition of *Current Procedural Terminology,* or CPT-4 for short. This book and its annual updates provide codes for nearly every treatment, test, and service a patient might receive.

These codes make medical information more standard, or uniform, than written descriptions. Medicare, Medicaid, and other health care plans require providers to use them. The use of ICD codes is required by HIPAA.

Some of the benefits of coding include:

- Coding ensures that the thousands of health care providers report the same conditions and procedures in exactly the same way.

- The collection of health information and statistics is more accurate.

- Medical reviews, or medical chart audits, are easier to perform. Medical chart audits can occur in both the physician's office and at the insurance company. The charts are reviewed for accuracy and appropriateness of codes used for claims.

- The processing of health insurance claims is more efficient and accurate.

Coding and Insurance

All codes you put on the form must be complete and correct. The CPT codes reported on a patient's insurance claim form determine what his or her health plan will pay. Insurers use

ICD codes to help determine **medical necessity.** This means the procedure or service being billed was reasonable for the patient's medical condition.

For example, an insurance company wouldn't consider a chest x-ray medically necessary if the ICD code was for an ear infection. But if the diagnostic code was for acute bronchitis, the insurance company probably would pay. The diagnosis code justifies the procedure code. On the other hand, inaccurate coding can lead to:

- delayed payment
- reduced payment
- denied payment

Of course, there also must be documentation in the patient's chart to support diagnoses and procedures that were coded correctly. You'll read more about the relationship between coding, chart documentation, and insurance later in this chapter and in Chapter 8.

Diagnostic Coding and the ICD-9

The ICD is a system of classifying diseases that was developed by the World Health Organization (WHO) in the 1930s and 1940s. The first ICD book was published in 1948. Since then, the list has been revised nine times. The latest revision, the ICD-10, has not yet been approved in United States. But it may be in the next few years. Until then, U.S. coders continue to use the ICD-9.

Closer Look

CODING ERRORS: EFFECTS ON PATIENTS

An insurance payment that is reduced or denied because of a coding error might create problems for the patient. But a wrong ICD code could cause the patient even bigger problems.

Suppose a patient comes in with a complaint of chest pain. Instead of coding "rule out myocardial infarction" (heart attack), you use the ICD code for "myocardial infarction" instead. This coding mistake might cause the patient to be labeled incorrectly in an insurance database as having heart disease. This could affect the patient's ability to get health, life, or disability insurance in the future.

The ICD-9-CM was published in the United States in 1979. It's updated each year, with codes being added, changed, and sometimes removed. The National Center for Health Statistics (NCHS), a U.S. government agency, keeps the list of diagnoses current.

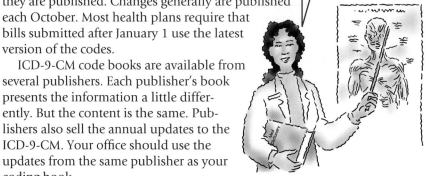

Coding requires a good knowledge of medical terms and anatomy. Keep reference materials handy in addition to your code book.

The WHO approves all changes before they are published. Changes generally are published each October. Most health plans require that bills submitted after January 1 use the latest version of the codes.

ICD-9-CM code books are available from several publishers. Each publisher's book presents the information a little differently. But the content is the same. Publishers also sell the annual updates to the ICD-9-CM. Your office should use the updates from the same publisher as your coding book.

The ICD-9-CM Code Book

The ICD-9-CM is made up of three volumes. They contain more than 10,000 diagnostic codes.

- *Volume 1: Tabular List of Diseases.* This book lists diseases in numerical order by their code numbers.
- *Volume 2: Alphabetic Index of Diseases.* This book contains diagnostic terms that don't appear in Volume 1.
- *Volume 3: Tabular List and Alphabetic Index of Procedures.* This book generally is used only by hospitals.

Closer Look   OFFICE FORMS AND CODE UPDATES

Remember to check your office's superbill and other forms that contain ICD or CPT codes each time they are updated. If any of the codes on the forms have changed, new forms must be printed.

Experts estimate that millions of dollars in insurance payments have been lost because an incorrect code was taken from an old office form that had not been updated.

Hospitals use Volume 3 to bill for the services and care they provide. Volumes 1 and 2 contain the diagnosis codes that justify physicians' services to patients. Those services will be billed by the physician's office, no matter where the services took place. For these reasons, we will look only at Volumes 1 and 2 in this chapter.

INSIDE VOLUME 1

Volume 1 organizes diseases and other conditions into 17 chapters, according to **etiology** (cause) or body system. The diseases are numbered in sequence within each chapter and throughout the book. These examples from the book's table of contents show how they are grouped.

- *Chapter 1: Infectious and Parasitic Diseases.* This chapter starts with disease 001 and goes to disease 139.

- *Chapter 7: Diseases of the Circulatory System.* The diseases in this chapter are numbered 390 to 459.

- *Chapter 8: Diseases of the Respiratory System.* This chapter contains diseases 460 to 519.

- *Chapter 9: Diseases of the Digestive System.* The diseases in this chapter begin at 520 and end at 579.

- *Chapter 17: Injury and Poisoning.* The conditions listed in this chapter are numbered 800 to 999.

As you can see, Chapters 1 and 17 group conditions according to what causes them. In Chapters 7 to 9, they are grouped according to the body system affected.

Each chapter is divided into *sections* of similar diseases. For example, the 139 diseases in Chapter 1 are organized into 16 sections, according to the type of disease. Three of these sections are:

- intestinal infectious diseases (001–009)

- viral diseases accompanied by exanthem (050–057)

- syphilis and other venereal diseases (090–099)

Disease Codes

Within each section, a three-digit code identifies each disease *category.* For example, in Chapter 1 the section of *viral diseases accompanied by exanthem* (a rash or skin eruption) is subdivided into these categories:

050	Smallpox
051	Cowpox and paravaccina
052	Chickenpox

053	Herpes zoster
054	Herpes simplex
055	Measles
056	Rubella
057	Other viral exanthemata

Fourth and Fifth Digits. Within each disease category, a fourth digit provides descriptions of its variations. In some cases, a fifth digit allows even more specifics. For example, here are *some* of the fourth and fifth digits you would have to choose from if you were coding a herpes simplex (054) diagnosis of a patient:

054.1	Genital herpes	
	054.10	Genital herpes, unspecified
	054.11	Herpetic vulvovaginitis
	054.12	Herpetic ulceration of vulva
	054.13	Herpetic infection of penis
	054.19	Other
054.2	Herpetic gingivostomatitis (cold sore on mouth)	
054.4	With ophthalmic (eye) complications	
	054.40	With unspecified ophthalmic complication
	054.41	Herpes simplex dermatitis of eyelid
	054.49	Other
054.7	With other specified complications	
054.8	With other unspecified complications	
054.9	With no mention of complication	

Codes and More Codes

Two lists of what are called "supplementary" classifications are also found in Volume 1.

- V-codes are used when a patient seeks care for something other than a current illness or injury.

- E-codes are used to explain the reason for an injury, but they must never be the primary code. Although they can be used with codes from any chapter, if appropriate, they are most often used with codes from Chapter 17.

Both lists of codes provide more information about the reason the patient was seen.

> Volume 1 tells you how many digits are needed to code each diagnosis correctly. In general, code to the most specific level available.

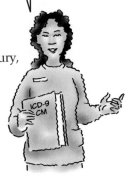

V-codes. V-codes all begin with the letter V. They range from V01 to V82. V-codes allow you to code a reason for a healthy patient's office visit. Perhaps the patient has come in for a vaccination (V03–V05) or for a routine physical exam (V70). None of the codes in the 17 chapters of Volume 1 would apply.

Here's another example of how V-codes are used. Suppose a patient once had a **malignant** (cancerous) **neoplasm** (tumor) of the stomach. Because of this past history, the patient needs regular checkups. You wouldn't code the reason for the visit as 230.2, neoplasm of the stomach. That code would mean the patient currently has the condition. Instead, you'd code the visit V10.04 (person history of malignant neoplasm of the stomach). This indicates that the patient once had a malignant neoplasm but doesn't have it now.

E-codes. E-codes range from E800 to E899. These codes are limited to one digit beyond the decimal point. But even so, they provide an amazing amount of detail. For example, suppose your office treats a patient who has broken his leg in a fall. For the diagnosis, you might code 822.1 (open fracture of patella). But here are just *some* of the choices you would have in coding how the injury happened:

E880	Fall on or from stairs or steps	
	E880.0	Escalator
	E880.1	Fall on or from sidewalk curb
	E880.9	Other stairs or steps
E881	Fall on or from ladder or scaffolding	
	E881.0	Fall from ladder
	E881.1	Fall from scaffolding
E882	Fall from or out of building or other structure	
E883	Fall into a hole or other opening in surface	
	E883.0	Accident from diving or jumping into water (swimming pool)
	E883.1	Accidental fall into well
	E883.2	Accidental fall into storm drain or manhole
	E883.9	Fall into other hole or other opening in surface
E884	Other fall from one level to another	
	E884.0	Fall from playground equipment
	E884.1	Fall from cliff
	E884.2	Fall from chair

	E884.3	Fall from wheelchair
	E884.4	Fall from bed
	E884.5	Fall from other furniture
	E884.6	Fall from commode (toilet)
	E884.9	Other fall from one level to another
E885		Fall on same level from slipping, tripping, or stumbling
	E885.0	Fall from (nonmotorized) scooter
	E885.1	Fall from roller skates/roller blades
	E885.2	Fall from skateboard
	E885.3	Fall from skis
	E885.4	Fall from snowboard
	E885.9	Fall from other slipping, tripping, or stumbling

Volume 1 Appendices

Volume 1 also contains four appendices, labeled A, C, D, and E. (Appendix B, a glossary of mental disorders, was removed from the ICD-9-CM in the 2006 edition.)

- Appendix A is used with Chapter 2 when coding neoplasms. Its M-codes identify the neoplasm's **morphology**, or form and structure. For example, the code M8070/3 shows that a tumor is a squamous cell carcinoma (M8070). The /3 indicates that it's the primary site of the cancer. M-codes are seldom used by physicians' offices.

- Appendix C provides the diagnostic codes to be used when a patient has a bad reaction to certain kinds of medications. For example, it tells you to code a patient's bad reaction to an antihistamine (in drug class 48:00) as 963.0 (poisoning by antiallergic and antiemetic drugs).

- Appendix D lists codes that describe equipment or materials responsible for a job-related injury or illness. For example, E919.4 (accident on woodworking machinery) would explain the diagnosis of 883.1 (complicated wound to fingers). Code 141 from Appendix D would further explain that this was a work injury from a circular saw.

- Appendix E is a list of all the three-digit categories in the ICD-9-CM.

Appendices A, C, and D are not used by Medicare or most other government programs. But they can be helpful in coding for other sources of payment.

INSIDE VOLUME 2

Volume 2 of the ICD-9-CM is divided into three sections.

- Section 1 is an alphabetic index of symptoms, diseases, and injuries. It's organized much differently than the classification system in Volume 1.

- Section 2 is a table of drugs and chemicals. It links each one to the code for its use in treatment, as well as to codes for various types of misuse.

- Section 3 is an alphabetic index of events that cause injury. This very detailed list is linked to the E-codes of Volume 1.

Alphabetic Index to Diseases and Injuries

You should always begin your coding of a diagnosis in this section—Section 1 of Volume 2. You should start with the condition and then the anatomical site. For example, if you were working with chest pain, you start with pain and then the body location.

This section is much more detailed than the lists of diseases in Volume 1. For example, if you look up *bleeding* in the index, here are a few of the entries you'll find under that main heading:

Bleeding (see also Hemorrhage) 459.0

anal 569.3

capillary 448.9

ear 388.69

following intercourse 626.7

gastrointestinal 578.9

gums 523.8

menopausal 627.0

nose 784.7

ovulation 626.6

postoperative 998.11

tendencies 286.9

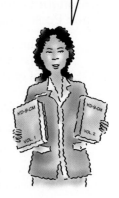

To be sure your codes are complete and correct, remember to use both Volumes 1 and 2.

Note that each entry is followed by a diagnostic code from Volume 1. This makes the index a better starting point than searching through Volume 1 for a likely section and disease category to fit the patient's condition.

You'd go from the index entry that best describes the patient's symptoms to the related code in Volume 1 and see if it's appropriate. Don't accept the code number in Volume 2 as the correct code without making this check.

Table of Drugs and Chemicals

This table in Section 2 of Volume 2 contains a long list of medicines, drugs, and other substances. It shows the code to assign
from Volume 1 when a patient is harmed by a drug or other
substance in each of these circumstances.

- *Accidental poisoning.* The patient received an accidental over-
  dose of the drug or was given or took the drug by mistake.
- *Therapeutic use.* The patient took or received the drug in the
  right dose to treat or prevent a disease.
- *Suicide attempt.* The patient took the drug in an effort to
  poison or injure himself.
- *Assault.* Someone gave the patient the drug in a deliberate
  attempt to harm him.
- *Undetermined.* It's not known whether the poisoning or
  injury from the drug was intended or accidental.

CODES FOR ASPIRIN

If you look up *aspirin* in the table, it provides the following codes.

- Poisoning 965.1
- Accidental E850.3
- Therapeutic Use E935.3
- Suicide E950.0
- Assault E962.0
- Undetermined E980.0

Alphabetic Index to External Cases of Injuries and Poisonings

This index in Section 3 of Volume 2 is much like the index to
diseases in Section 1. It leads you to codes that describe causes
of injuries, accidents, and violence. The main entries in this
index are usually a type of accident or violence, such as *Assault,
Collision,* or *Fall.* Here's an example from the index.

Assault (homicidal) (by) (in) E968.9

air gun E968.6

acid E961

swallowed E962.1

BB gun E968.6

bite NEC E968.8

   of human being E968.7

bomb ((placed in) car or house) E965.8

   antipersonnel E965.5

   letter E965.7

   petrol E965.6

brawl (hand) (fists) (foot) E960.0

cut, any part of body E966

dagger E966

explosives E965.9

   bomb (see also Assault, bomb) E965.8

   dynamite E965.8

fight (hand) (Fists) (foot) E960.0

   with weapon E968.9

     blunt or thrown E968.2

     cutting or piercing E966

     firearm—see Shooting, homicide

You use Section 3 just like you use Section 1. You find the cause of the injury in this index and it tells you the related E-code to assign.

Remember that E-codes aren't diagnosis codes. They give details about the condition, but they shouldn't be used in place of the diagnosis code. For example, you'd give a patient who fractured her tibia in a fall off a curb a code of 823.80 (fracture of tibia, closed) from Chapter 17 of Volume 1. You would add the code E880.1 to report that the fall was off a curb. The E880.1 would never appear alone without a diagnosis code.

Coding Medical Diagnoses

The Hands On procedure on page 264 provides a step-by-step guide to performing diagnostic coding. The procedures are drawn from guidelines developed by CMS for submitting claims to Medicare. Some private insurance companies may have different requirements, but most have adopted the CMS standards. Following them should satisfy most third-party payers.

You'll now read some added information that will help you when following the Hands On procedure. These tips also will help you better understand and use the ICD-9-CM to code the patient's diagnosis.

THE MAIN TERM RULE

As the Hands On procedure indicates, the first step in coding a diagnosis is to locate the main term in the diagnosis statement. This will usually appear on the superbill, fee slip, or encounter form, where the physician will have either checked it off or written it in. Another source is the progress notes in the patient's medical chart. The diagnosis usually will be listed there as the *impression*. The *main term rule* is that you look for the *main term* in the diagnosis or description.

Applying the Main Term Rule. For example, if the diagnosis is malignant hypertension, the main term would be *hypertension*. That is the term you'd look up in the alphabetic index of Volume 2 when you begin the coding process. Under *hypertension*, you'll find all the different types of hypertension listed. *Malignant* will be one of the types.

Closer Look   EXCEPTIONS TO THE MAIN TERM RULE

Keep these exceptions to the *main term rule* in mind when you use the alphabetic index in Volume 2 of the ICD-9-CM.

1. Obstetric conditions may be found under these main terms:
   - *delivery*
   - *pregnancy*
   - *puerperal*

2. Complications of medical or surgical procedures can be found under *complication*.

3. V-codes are found under main entries such as:
   - *admissions*
   - *examination*
   - *history of observation*
   - *problem* (with)
   - *status*
   - *vaccination*
   - *encounter for*
   - *follow-up*

You take the code next to *malignant* in Volume 2 and find it in the tabular list in Volume 1. Turn to the chapter in Volume 1 that contains the code number and look for the code. You'd then choose the specific code from the choices listed.

What Diagnosis to Use

Since the diagnosis can change from visit to visit, you always must go with the most current visit. Sometimes what's thought to be the diagnosis on one visit can change on the next visit. By then, test results would be back and the diagnosis could turn out to be something else.

It's also acceptable to code the symptoms if there's no definite diagnosis. For example, suppose a patient comes to the office with stomach pains and nausea. If the doctor cannot make a definite diagnosis without blood tests or x-rays, you would code the stomach pains and the nausea instead.

Primary Codes

A patient will have a **primary diagnosis** on each visit to the office. This is simply the patient's chief complaint or the reason he sought medical attention that day. The code for that diagnosis, complaint, or reason is the *primary code* for the visit.

The primary code is always listed first on the insurance claim form. In most cases this will be a CMS-1500, the standard form that Medicare and most insurance companies use. You can see a sample CMS-1500 containing a primary code and other coded information on page 246.

MULTIPLE CODES

Although each visit has a primary code, you may have to code other diagnoses as well. When patients have more than one diagnosis, the insurance company may need an accurate picture of the patient's total condition. This is especially true if a condition unrelated to the visit affects the patient's treatment. Here's how that might happen.

Suppose a patient has the following active conditions and diagnoses:

- type II diabetes
- degenerative arthritis
- hypertension
- pernicious anemia

Today, however, she has come to the office seeking treatment for the flu. Her primary diagnosis for this visit is the reason for

PLEASE
DO NOT
STAPLE
IN THIS
AREA

CARRIER

HEALTH INSURANCE CLAIM FORM

| | PICA | | PICA | |

1. MEDICARE	MEDICAID	CHAMPUS	CHAMPVA	GROUP HEALTH PLAN	FECA BLK LUNG	OTHER	1a. INSURED'S I.D. NUMBER (FOR PROGRAM IN ITEM 1)
X (Medicare #)	(Medicaid #)	(Sponsor's SSN)	(VA File #)	(SSN or ID)	(SSN)	(ID)	000-00-0000A

2. PATIENT'S NAME (Last Name, First Name, Middle Initial)	3. PATIENT'S BIRTH DATE MM DD YY	SEX	4. INSURED'S NAME (Last Name, First Name, Middle Initial)
Naomi A Dishman	04 14 24	M [] F [X]	Same

5. PATIENT'S ADDRESS (No., Street)	6. PATIENT RELATIONSHIP TO INSURED	7. INSURED'S ADDRESS (No., Street)
405 Carolina Ave	Self [] Spouse [] Child [] Other []	

CITY	STATE	8. PATIENT STATUS	CITY	STATE
Danville	VA	Single [] Married [X] Other []		

ZIP CODE	TELEPHONE (Include Area Code)		ZIP CODE	TELEPHONE (INCLUDE AREA CODE)
24540	(434) 555-5555	Employed [] Full-Time Student [] Part-Time Student []		( )

9. OTHER INSURED'S NAME (Last Name, First Name, Middle Initial)	10. IS PATIENT'S CONDITION RELATED TO:	11. INSURED'S POLICY GROUP OR FECA NUMBER
NONE		

a. OTHER INSURED'S POLICY OR GROUP NUMBER	a. EMPLOYMENT? (CURRENT OR PREVIOUS) YES [] NO [X]	a. INSURED'S DATE OF BIRTH MM DD YY SEX M [] F []
b. OTHER INSURED'S DATE OF BIRTH MM DD YY SEX M [] F []	b. AUTO ACCIDENT? PLACE (State) YES [] NO [X]	b. EMPLOYER'S NAME OR SCHOOL NAME
c. EMPLOYER'S NAME OR SCHOOL NAME	c. OTHER ACCIDENT? YES [X] NO []	c. INSURANCE PLAN NAME OR PROGRAM NAME
d. INSURANCE PLAN NAME OR PROGRAM NAME	10d. RESERVED FOR LOCAL USE	d. IS THERE ANOTHER HEALTH BENEFIT PLAN? YES [] NO [] If yes, return to and complete item 9 a-d.

READ BACK OF FORM BEFORE COMPLETING & SIGNING THIS FORM.

12. PATIENT'S OR AUTHORIZED PERSON'S SIGNATURE I authorize the release of any medical or other information necessary to process this claim. I also request payment of government benefits either to myself or to the party who accepts assignment below.

SIGNED Signature on File   DATE 052803

13. INSURED'S OR AUTHORIZED PERSON'S SIGNATURE I authorize payment of medical benefits to the undersigned physician or supplier for services described below.

SIGNED

14. DATE OF CURRENT: ILLNESS (First symptom) OR INJURY (Accident) OR PREGNANCY(LMP) MM DD YY 05 28 03	15. IF PATIENT HAS HAD SAME OR SIMILAR ILLNESS. GIVE FIRST DATE MM DD YY	16. DATES PATIENT UNABLE TO WORK IN CURRENT OCCUPATION MM DD YY FROM TO MM DD YY
17. NAME OF REFERRING PHYSICIAN OR OTHER SOURCE	17a. I.D. NUMBER OF REFERRING PHYSICIAN	18. HOSPITALIZATION DATES RELATED TO CURRENT SERVICES MM DD YY FROM TO MM DD YY
19. RESERVED FOR LOCAL USE		20. OUTSIDE LAB? YES [] NO [] $ CHARGES

21. DIAGNOSIS OR NATURE OF ILLNESS OR INJURY. (RELATE ITEMS 1,2,3 OR 4 TO ITEM 24E BY LINE)

1. 845.03
2. 250.00
3.
4.

22. MEDICAID RESUBMISSION CODE   ORIGINAL REF. NO.

23. PRIOR AUTHORIZATION NUMBER

24. A. DATE(S) OF SERVICE From MM DD YY	To MM DD YY	B. Place of Service	C. Type of Service	D. PROCEDURES, SERVICES, OR SUPPLIES (Explain Unusual Circumstances) CPT/HCPCS	MODIFIER	E. DIAGNOSIS CODE	F. $ CHARGES	G. DAYS OR UNITS	H. EPSDT Family Plan	I. EMG	J. COB	K. RESERVED FOR LOCAL USE
05 28 03	05 28 03	11		99213		1	100 00	1				
05 28 03	05 28 03	11		82947		2	25 00	1				

25. FEDERAL TAX I.D. NUMBER SSN EIN	26. PATIENT'S ACCOUNT NO.	27. ACCEPT ASSIGNMENT? (For govt. claims, see back)	28. TOTAL CHARGE	29. AMOUNT PAID	30. BALANCE DUE
54-0000000 [] []	1234	[X] YES [] NO	$ 125 00	$	$ 125 00

31. SIGNATURE OF PHYSICIAN OR SUPPLIER INCLUDING DEGREES OR CREDENTIALS (I certify that the statements on the reverse apply to this bill and are made a part thereof.) SIGNED DATE	32. NAME AND ADDRESS OF FACILITY WHERE SERVICES WERE RENDERED (If other than home or office)	33. PHYSICIAN'S, SUPPLIER'S BILLING NAME, ADDRESS, ZIP CODE & PHONE # JOSEPH G NORTH, MD 1111 GRAYSON STREET DANVILLE VA PIN# GRP#

(APPROVED BY AMA COUNCIL ON MEDICAL SERVICE 8/88)   **PLEASE PRINT OR TYPE**

APPROVED OMB-0938-0008 FORM CMS-1500 (12-90), FORM RRB-1500,
APPROVED OMB-1215-0055 FORM OWCP-1500, APPROVED OMB-0720-0001 (CHAMPUS)

PATIENT AND INSURED INFORMATION

PHYSICIAN OR SUPPLIER INFORMATION

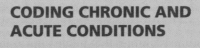

Running Smoothly

CODING CHRONIC AND ACUTE CONDITIONS

What if you have to code a condition that's both chronic and acute?

Mr. Jones has a long history of asthma and bronchitis. Each spring, the pollen makes his breathing problems worse. You're not sure whether to code his diagnosis as chronic or acute when he seeks treatment at such times.

Respiratory diseases and orthopedic conditions tend to be both chronic (continuing) and acute (temporarily severe). If there are separate categories for chronic and acute in the disease category, use both. List the code for the acute problem first, since that's the reason for his visit. Then, list the code for the underlying chronic condition.

her appointment—symptoms of the flu. Since she has diabetes, however, she always should see a doctor when she has the flu. Her diabetes also will affect how the doctor treats her influenza.

Therefore, you would code the diagnosis of type II diabetes below the primary code on the CMS-1500. This information tells the insurance company the visit was necessary and the treatment was appropriate. Without it, the insurance company might deny payment on the basis that the visit or treatment was medically unnecessary.

Late Effects

Late effects are conditions that result from a past injury or illness. They are present long after treatment for the injury or illness has ended. For example, patients who have in the past suffered a cerebrovascular accident (CVA), or stroke, may have effects that linger after their recovery.

For instance, a patient may have a diagnosis of left hemiparesis (paralysis) as a result of a stroke three years earlier. For this patient's visit, you would code the current condition—left hemiparesis—first, as the primary diagnosis. It would be the primary code. The code number identifying the cause—that is, the original illness or injury—would come second.

THE CONNECTION BETWEEN LATE EFFECTS CODES AND THE ORIGINAL ILLNESS OR INJURY

Here are some examples that might appear in the diagnosis section of a CMS-1500. They will help you see the relationship between late effects codes and the original illness or injury coded second. So you can tell what each code means, descriptions have been added in parenthesis.

1. 905.4 (late effect of fracture of lower extremities)

2. 821.1 (open fracture of patella)

1. 137.3 (late effects of tuberculosis of bones and joints)

2. 015.14 (tuberculosis of hip, tubercle bacilli found by bacterial culture)

1. 139.0 (late effects of viral encephalitis)

2. 062.9 (mosquito-borne viral encephalitis, unspecified)

The physician's notes on the visit in the patient's medical record often will provide clues to whether a late effects code should be used. Here are some key words to look for.

- late
- due to an old injury
- due to a previous illness
- sequela of
- resulting from

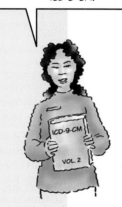

If you're looking for the correct late effect codes, a good place to start is under "Late" in the alphabetic index of Volume 2 of the ICD-9-CM.

CODING SUSPECTED CONDITIONS

In hospitals, medical coders don't list patients' diagnoses until testing is complete. In other words, they code from complete information. In a medical office, you'll have to report the reason for the patient's visit when it occurs. You'll be limited by the information available at the time. Often, this will be only the patient's complaint and the physician's best guess about what is causing it. The physician may write *probable,* or *rule out* along with his suspected diagnosis. However, you cannot code this diagnosis as the reason for the visit until it's confirmed.

You don't want to put in the patient's record that he has a condition he may not really have. Instead, you should code the reason the patient came in. That reason could be:

- a test result that was abnormal
- a sign or a symptom
- any reason the patient thought he should be seen

> A popular—and proper—saying among professional coders is: _Don't code what's not there._

Here's an example. A patient makes an appointment because he's been having severe headaches. The physician suspects a brain tumor and schedules the patient for an MRI (magnetic resonance imaging) of his head. The physician writes _rule out brain tumor_ in the patient's chart. But you can't code the diagnosis as _brain tumor_ until the MRI test confirms it. You don't have that information on this visit. If it is coded as a brain tumor, this inaccurate information will follow the patient around for the rest of his life.

Signs, Symptoms, and Chapter 16

Fortunately, the ICD-9-CM provides the solution for this problem. Chapter 16 in Volume 1 is titled Symptoms, Signs, and Ill-Defined Conditions. Categories 780–789 contain detailed lists of symptoms for each part of the body. You should use this section to code the patient's symptoms until a diagnosis is confirmed.

Category 784 is "Symptoms involving head and neck." Within this category, code 784.0 identifies "Headache: facial pain or pain in head (NOS)." (NOS means _not otherwise specified_.) This would be the primary code for the first visit. On the second visit, the MRI results are back. They confirm a glioma (a type of cancerous tumor) in the frontal lobe.

Following the alphabetic index in Volume 2 to the numerical list of diseases in Volume 1 will guide you in converting this diagnosis into the proper diagnostic code. As long as the patient is being seen for this problem, from this visit on, 191.1 (malignant neoplasm of brain, frontal lobe) will be the primary code.

ICD-9-CM CONVENTIONS

Conventions are rules that apply to using the ICD-9-CM. They help direct the user to the proper code and always should be followed strictly. Conventions can take several forms.

- general notes using specific terms
- cross-references
- abbreviations
- use of punctuation marks
- use of symbols
- different types of treatments
- changes in format

Major Conventions in the ICD-9-CM

Convention	Meaning	Example
braces { }	Each term on the open side of the brace is incomplete without the term on the closed side of the brace.	478.1 Other diseases of nasal cavity and sinuses Abscess
parentheses ( )	Parentheses enclose words that may be present or absent in the diagnosis statement without affecting the code to be used.	Necrosis } of nose (septum) Ulcer
NEC	"Not elsewhere classifiable"; should be used only when there's not enough information to code more specifically	Infection Streptococcal NEC 041.00 Group A 041.01 B 041.02 As soon as bacterium is identified, code for specific infection.
NOS	"Not otherwise specified"; tells the coder to look for a more specific code	007.9 Unspecified protozoal intestinal disease Flagellate diarrhea Protozoal dysentery NOS
INCLUDES	Modifies, further defines, or gives more examples of the content of a category	477 Allergic rhinitis INCLUDES Allergic rhinitis (seasonal) (nonseasonal) Hay fever
EXCLUDES	Tells the coder to not use the code for this condition and directs coder to the proper code	EXCLUDES Allergic rhinitis with asthma (bronchial) (493.0)
see see also see category	These phrases direct the coder to other places to consider. These instructions ALWAYS should be followed.	Itch (see also Pruritus) 698.9
use additional code	Tells the coder to add another code to further explain the diagnosis	438.6 Alterations of sensations Use additional code to identify the altered sensation.
code first underlying disease	Tells the coder to code the underlying disease that caused the current problem as well	321.3 Meningitis due to trypanosomiasis Code first underlying disease (086.0–086.9).

Some of the common conventions are included in the table shown above. Each publisher of the ICD-9-CM uses these conventions. Many add even more conventions of their own to assist coders in using their books.

The CPT-4 Code Book

The CPT-4 is the fourth edition of *Current Procedural Terminology*. The book lists common medical procedures and services and a code for each one. It was first published by the American Medical Association in 1966. The fourth edition was published in

1977. That was the last major revision of the book, but it's updated every year.

A CPT code is a five-digit numeric code for a specific medical procedure or supply that a physician provides to a patient. Here's an example of some codes. Notice how they are listed in relation to each other.

27556	Open treatment of knee dislocation, with or without internal or external fixation; without primary ligamentous repair or augmentation/reconstruction
27557	with primary ligamentous repair
27558	with primary ligamentous repair, with augmentation/reconstruction
27660	Closed treatment of patellar dislocation; without anesthesia
	(For recurrent dislocation, see 27420–27424)
27562	requiring anesthesia
	(27564 has been deleted. To report, see 27560, 27562, 27566)
27566	Open treatment of patellar dislocation, with or without partial or total patellectomy

As you can see, the CPT-4 codes are organized much like the ICD-9 codes. There's a main code that describes a procedure. Listed under it are other codes with indented descriptions of variations of the main procedure. CPT codes just don't have decimal points like ICD-9 codes do.

Another difference is that some CPT codes can have modifiers. You'll read more about modifiers later in this chapter.

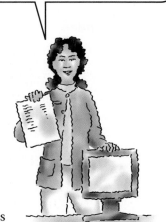

Remember, if your office uses a superbill, you must review it yearly when the CPT codes are updated, just as you do with the ICD-9 codes. Computer billing software may have to be updated too.

INSIDE THE CPT-4

The CPT codes are divided into six sections. Like the chapters in Volume 1 of the ICD-9-CM, the codes in each section of the CPT-4 are listed by number. The diagnostic codes are organized by etiology or body system, however, while the CPT codes are organized by the type of service. The six sections of the CPT-4 are:

- *Evaluation and Management.* These are the codes used to charge for office visits. All codes in this section begin with the number 9.

- *Anesthesia.* These codes are organized according to body site (head, thorax, hip, etc.). Then, under each body site, the specific procedure is listed. These codes all begin with 0.

- *Surgery.* Surgery codes begin with numbers 1 through 6. Like the anesthesia codes, they are organized according to which part of the body is involved.

- *Radiology.* All radiology codes begin with the number 7. Radiology procedures generally aren't done in a physician's office, however.

- *Pathology and Laboratory.* This section includes every lab test that can be ordered. These codes all begin with 8.

- *Medicine.* These codes cover nonsurgical treatments and services that ordinarily take place in a doctor's office (injections, blood pressure checks, etc.). They all begin with a 9, just like the Evaluation and Management codes.

CPT-4 SECTION GUIDELINES

Each section begins with a set of guidelines for coding the kinds of procedures listed in that particular section. Pay close attention to these guidelines. They contain much useful information.

- definitions and explanations to assist the coder
- a list of procedures new to the section
- modifiers that can be used with the section's codes
- codes to use when an unlisted procedure is performed
- directions on how to file a special report

The Index

The final part of the CPT-4 is an index that lists every procedure alphabetically. You use this index much like you use the alphabetic index in Volume 2 of the ICD-9-CM. That is, you look up the procedure in the CPT index first and then find the number it gives in the lists of codes.

The Hands On feature on page 265 provides a step-by-step process for assigning procedure codes. You'll get tips for using specific kinds of codes later in this chapter.

HCPCS

The CPT codes don't include codes for many kinds of medical services that are not provided by a physician. Some of these missing services include:

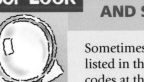

UNLISTED PROCEDURES AND SPECIAL REPORTS

Sometimes a physician will perform a service that's not listed in the CPT-4 book. The book provides unlisted codes at the beginning of each section to use when such a procedure is done. When you use an unlisted code, you also must submit a special report with the claim form. This report is usually in the form of a letter and should include the following information:

- explanation of the need for the procedure
- description of its nature and extent
- the time, effort, and equipment needed
- complexity of symptoms
- final diagnosis
- physical findings
- diagnostic and therapeutic procedures
- concurrent problems
- follow-up care

- ambulance service
- wheelchairs
- orthotics (devices to assist a weakened limb)
- hearing and vision services

As a result, CMS developed another coding system in the 1980s to provide codes for such items. This system is the Healthcare Common Procedure Coding System, or HCPCS (called *hick picks* by health care professionals). Physicians must use HCPCS codes when billing for services and supplies provided to patients covered by Medicare or Medicaid.

Outpatient surgery centers must use the codes when reporting charges for any patient who receives health benefits sponsored by the federal government. This requirement also applies to hospitals that perform outpatient surgery.

There are two levels of HCPCS codes.

- Level 1 codes are included in the CPT-4 lists. They are used with Level 2 codes to provide greater detail about services and supplies.

- Level 2 codes are five-digit codes that begin with the letter A to V, followed by a four-digit number. For example,

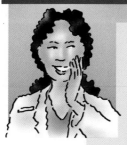

Secrets for Success

USING MEDICAL TERMS: INPATIENTS AND OUTPATIENTS

You'll hear the terms *inpatient* and *outpatient* often in your career in health care. By using their prefixes—*in* and *out*—it's easy to remember the difference.

- An *inpatient* is a patient who is *in* the hospital.
- An *outpatient* is a patient who is *out of* (not in) the hospital.

Hospitals provide services to outpatients too. But the difference is that these patients don't stay in the hospital overnight. If they did, they'd become inpatients!

L8100 is the code for an elastic support stocking, ending below the knee and of medium weight.

The list of Level 2 codes comes out once a year in the *National Coding Manual*. This book can be ordered from the American Hospital Association, the AMA, or other publishers of the CPT-4 code book.

Coding Services and Procedures

Although the Hands On procedure on page 265 tells you how to use the CPT-4, each section's codes must be treated a little differently. It's helpful to know the basics about each type of codes, even if you never work in that kind of office. Here are some tips and examples for using each type.

EVALUATION AND MANAGEMENT CODES

The Evaluation and Management (E/M) codes are used to charge for the patient's visit with the physician. That visit can take place in any number of places. Here are just some of the possible settings for a patient visit.

- office
- hospital room
- hospital emergency room
- patient's home
- nursing home
- rehabilitation facility

Basically, each E/M code measures the physician's level of involvement with the patient. This can range from a short visit that deals with a single, simple problem to a longer visit in which the physician deals with several problems that are difficult or severe.

Selecting an E/M Code

It's always the physician's job to decide which E/M code to assign to a visit. However, you should know what each requires to support the assigning of that code. That way, you can be sure the chart information supports the code and the billing will be correct.

All E/M codes are based on these seven factors.

1. history
2. physical examination
3. medical decision making
4. nature of the presenting problem
5. counseling the patient or a family member
6. time—the length of the visit
7. coordination of care with other providers

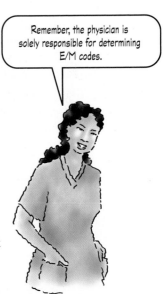

Remember, the physician is solely responsible for determining E/M codes.

The first three factors are **key components.** The rest are contributing factors in determining the level of the visit.

All three key components must be present to assign an E/M code to a new patient visit. For current or "established" patients, two key components are required. In general, they also determine how high a level of E/M code can be assigned.

THE ANESTHESIA AND SURGERY CODES

The anesthesia codes and the surgery codes are closely related in these ways.

- Both are organized by the place on the body being treated.
- Both are then subdivided by the procedure being performed on that part of the body.
- Both are coded by medical office staff even if the procedure takes place in a hospital.

The anesthesia section of the CPT-4 uses two types of **modifiers.** These are letters or numbers that are added to a code to provide more detail. One anesthesia modifier is a standard type that is found in all sections of the CPT. The other type is a special

Closer Look

CODING REFERRALS AND CONSULTATIONS

There are four categories of consultations.

- office
- initial inpatient
- follow-up inpatient
- confirmatory

Each category has its own reporting instructions.

When a physician asks another provider for advice about a specific problem, the second provider becomes a consultant. The initial encounter is coded as a consultation. The documentation must support this.

- A letter must accompany the patient seeing the consultant.
- The consultant must send a letter back to the first physician outlining the findings.

If the consultant takes over part or all of the patient's care, follow-ups are coded as regular visits.

A confirmatory consultation is considered a second opinion.

- The consultant offers only an opinion and advice.
- A confirmatory consultant does not take over treatment of the patient.

---

physical status modifier. It's a two-digit code that begins with the letter P and ends in a number from 1 to 6.

The physical status modifier tells the patient's condition at the time anesthesia was administered. It helps determine the difficulty of the service the anesthesiologist performed. For example, a P1 modifier shows the anesthesia was given to a normal, healthy patient. A P5 modifier indicates a patient who was not expected to survive without the procedure.

CPT SURGICAL PACKAGES

Many surgical procedures are coded as a surgical package. Included in the package (and the CPT code) are:

- after the surgery has been decided upon, there can be one related E/M meeting immediately before or on the day of the surgery to gather history and other information

- administration of local anesthesia
- the operation itself
- normal follow-up care after the operation

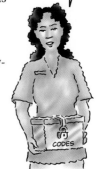

Remember, services that are combined in a surgical package can't be coded and billed separately.

These different components are bundled together and included in a single code. As long as the surgery goes as planned, there is no need for additional codes. Any procedures to deal with these complications should be coded separately.

Some insurance companies have a set number of follow-up days for care after surgery. Find out what these limits are so that you can bill for any extra hospital, office, or other outpatient visits. Also, the surgical package only includes follow-up care directly related to the recovery from the procedure itself and not related conditions.

Surgical Codes and Medicare. CMS defines surgical packages for Medicare patients differently than other insurers. According to CMS, complications that don't require a revisit to the operating room are included in the price of the surgery.

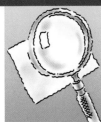

Closer Look   CODING INPATIENT SERVICES

Most of the coding in a medical office will be for outpatients. But some of your coding work may be for inpatients. This is because hospitals only bill for services they provide.

For example, if a patient is hospitalized for surgery, the hospital will bill for the patient's room and meals, nursing care, the use of the operating room and recovery room, and so on. But its bill won't include the surgeon's or anesthesiologist's services.

Medical office coders are concerned only with the physician's services, no matter where they are performed. So if a physician from your office examines or treats a patient in the hospital, you'll code these services and submit the charges for them on a CMS-1500 (universal claim form).

Basically, billing is determined by who provides the service, not by where it's performed. That's why you may be coding services that take place outside your medical office.

Other Surgical Coding Tips

Here are some other things you should know about using the surgical codes in the CPT-4.

- *The integumentary system.* This section of surgical codes has codes for which a measurement is needed. The size of the defect and the size of the specimen both must be measured before they are sent to the lab for testing. All codes listed in this section include simple closure.

- *Repairs.* The CPT-4 defines three types of repairs—simple, intermediate, and complex. Repairs should be measured in centimeters so they can be coded properly.

- *Cast reapplication.* You can't assign the same code to replacing a cast as you did to the original cast application. That's because the original code includes treatment of the fracture; replacing the cast does not. Therefore, the replacement code carries a lower payment rate.

- *Multiple procedures on the same day.* Code these procedures separately unless they are part of a package. They should be coded on the claim form in order, from major procedures to minor ones.

THE RADIOLOGY CODES

The radiology section of the CPT-4 is divided into four parts to match the four main types of radiology services.

- diagnostic radiology (diagnostic imaging)
- diagnostic ultrasound
- radiation oncology (radiation therapy)
- nuclear medicine

Within each part, the codes generally are arranged by anatomic site—from the top of the body to the bottom. Many codes indicate the number of views in a particular test. That's because the more views there are, the greater the costs for film, developing, and the technician's time.

Some radiology tests require that a contrast medium be used. This is a liquid that's administered to the patient to enhance the image on the film. The codes for these tests indicate either *with contrast* or *without contrast.* Here's how to assign the correct code.

- If the contrast medium is given intravascularly (injected into the bloodstream), code the test *with contrast.*

- If the contrast medium is given orally or rectally, use the test code for *without contrast.*

If the same physician performs, supervises, and interprets the procedure, two codes should be used. For example, the physician may inject the contrast medium, supervise the test, and interpret the results.

The code for the procedure can be found in the surgery, radiology, or medicine section. The code for supervision and interpretation is found in the radiology section. The physician must put a written report in the patient's medical record in order to bill this second code.

If two physicians are involved in the procedure—for example, a surgeon and a radiologist—the radiology portion is billed by the radiologist.

PATHOLOGY AND LABORATORY CODES

These codes are divided into several sections that include:

- drug testing
- panels of tests
- chemistry testing
- antibody testing
- urinalysis
- consultations with pathologists

The pathology and laboratory section contains codes for just about every blood test and combination of tests a physician might order. The last part of the section includes services and procedures provided by a pathologist. These include:

- gross (can be seen by the naked eye) examination of tissue removed during surgery
- examination by microscope of tissue removed during surgery
- postmortem examination or autopsy

Each tissue specimen is submitted under a different identifying code for diagnosis by the pathologist. The codes represent the level of the physician's work. The CPT-4 also provides codes for reporting postmortem exams and autopsies.

Automated Multichannel Tests

A subsection of the lab section contains codes for automated multichannel tests. These are blood chemistry tests that are often ordered in combination by the physician. The samples are analyzed together by machine in the lab.

A long list of blood tests falls into this category. When any two or more of them are performed on a patient, they can't be coded separately. Instead you must code and bill for them under a special automated multichannel test code. The code number you assign depends on the number of tests from the list that were performed. For example:

- 80004 means four tests from the list were performed.
- 80012 means 12 tests from the list were performed
- 80016 means between 13 and 16 tests from the list were performed.
- 80018 means 17 to 18 tests from the list were performed.
- 80019 means 19 tests from the list were performed.

When the physician orders blood tests on a patient, make sure they are all on the list before you assign a single code. Any that are not on the list must be coded individually.

CODING AUTOMATED MULTICHANNEL TESTS

Here's an example. Suppose the lab performs these three tests for a patient:

- bilirubin, total and direct (82251)
- cholesterol (82465)
- blood urea nitrogen (BUN) (84520)

Since all these tests are on the list of automated multichannel tests, you would not use the three individual codes shown above. Instead, you would code them 80003, the code for performing three automated multichannel tests.

But suppose the physician had ordered a blood acetaldehyde test (82000) instead of the BUN. Blood acetaldehyde is not on the list of automated multichannel tests. In this case you would code 80002, for two automated multichannel tests (bilirubin and cholesterol), and code the blood acetaldehyde test separately.

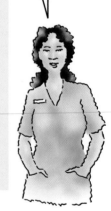

Remember, treat automated multichannel tests like surgical packages. You can't bill each test separately.

USING THE MEDICINE CODES

Like the other five sections of the CPT-4 book, this section includes guidelines for proper coding. Pay special attention to the information about coding immunizations. These codes include numbers 90701 to 90749 in the CPT.

Immunization injections usually are given when the patient comes to the office for a routine physical exam, or for some minor problem. When an immunization injection is given at such times, use two codes—one for the visit and the other for the injection.

For example, suppose a patient with controlled hypertension (high blood pressure) comes into the office for a blood pressure check. He's examined briefly by a nurse or medical assistant while the physician is in the office. Then he's given a polio immunization. Here's how you would code this visit. The CPT description that follows each code is included only to help you understand the example.

1. 99211—office and other outpatient visit for the evaluation and management of an established patient, which may not require the presence of a physician. Usually, the presenting problems are minimal. Typically, five minutes are spent performing or supervising services. (This code generally is used for examination by employees of the practice while a physician is in the office but not performing the examination.)

2. 90713—poliomyelitis vaccine

For therapeutic or diagnostic injections (codes 90782–90799), you also must identify what was injected (90281–90399). For example, in the CPT-4, the code 90782 is for *therapeutic injection of medication (specify); subcutaneous or transmuscular.* This code is the same for a number of injectable substances. This makes the additional code identifying the substance necessary.

OTHER GUIDELINES FOR INJECTION CODES

Here are some other guidelines for using the injection codes.

- A code for giving the injection (90471–90472) should be added.
- If a separate service was performed that was significant, the appropriate E/M code also should be reported.

If you'll be billing Medicare, the cost of giving injections is included in the charge for the visit. You may, however, bill a separate charge for the drug itself. So the drug administered should be coded separately in this case too.

The medicine section also contains codes for a wide range of other services. This includes codes for cardiac diagnostic tests, such as EKGs and echocardiograms. It even provides codes for home healthcare and performing CPR.

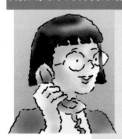

Q: *I think coding diagnoses and procedures is probably the hardest part of my job as a medical assistant. There's just so much to consider! I know my office manager doesn't like having insurance claims delayed or rejected because they were coded poorly. How can I become a better coder?*

A: Never guess if you're unsure how to code something! You can ask the office manager, the physician, or another staff member who knows about using the ICD-9 and CPT-4.

The American Medical Association (AMA) publishes books to help coders do their job. It also publishes *CPT Assistant,* a magazine written by CPT experts. The magazine contains articles designed to make coding easier. It also will keep you up to date on coding changes.

The AMA and many other organizations offer classes, workshops, and online training on medical coding. The AMA's Web site at www.ama-assn.org also contains helpful information about the CPT-4 and ICD-9 codes.

CPT DOS AND DON'TS

Here are some final tips for becoming a good medical coder.

- Always use the latest edition of the CPT.
- Refer to guidelines in each section regularly. Don't expect to know all the guidelines from memory. It can't be done!
- Make sure diagnosis codes clearly support CPT codes on the claim form. But *never* change an ICD code just to accomplish this.
- Never hesitate to ask the physician to clarify a code, procedure, or chart documentation.
- Know the CPT modifiers and use them when appropriate.

CPT Modifiers

Each section of the CPT-4 contains two-digit numbers known as modifiers. These modifiers allow coders to provide more information about the service being billed. For example:

- The surgery modifier 20 indicates that the physician used an operating microscope to perform the surgery.
- The surgery modifier 62 reveals that two physicians performed this procedure.

- The surgery modifier 76 reports that this is a repeat procedure by the same physician.
- The anesthesia modifier 23 signifies that anesthesia was used in a procedure that normally would not require it.

There are several ways to write modifiers.

- Write the five-digit CPT code followed by a hyphen and then the two-digit modifier. (for example, 28702-22)

Legal Brief   CODING AND FRAUD

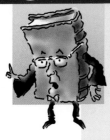

The Health Insurance Portability and Accountability Act of 1996 (HIPAA) defines fraud as *an intentional deception or misrepresentation . . . that could result in an unauthorized payment.* It's important to note that the mere act of filing a false claim is fraud, whether payment is made or not.

To combat fraud, CMS hires outside organizations to randomly review Medicare claims and compare them to the medical records of those patients. Many private insurance companies and state insurance departments also have units to combat fraud.

In medical coding, the most common examples of fraud are upcoding and unbundling.

- **Upcoding** is submitting a code for a service the physician hasn't performed. This often involves coding a service related to but more complex (and thus more expensive) than what was actually provided.

- **Unbundling** is submitting a code for each piece of a service package, instead of the single code for the entire package. Its goal is to gain greater payment by charging for each service separately.

Insurance examiners will downcode if your documentation differs from your code's description. This means they'll reimburse for a less costly service. .

Medicare has the same authority as the Internal Revenue Service (IRS) to audit your office's financial records. This means the claims you code and submit could be audited months or years after payment has been received.

The bottom line on fraud is don't do it! Not only is it illegal and the penalties severe, but submitting a false claim is a violation of your professional ethics as a medical assistant.

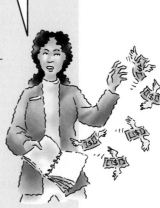

- Write the code without a hyphen separating it from the modifier. (for example, 2870222)
- If more than one modifier is needed, use the hyphen after the five-digit code, followed by 99 and then the modifiers. (for example, 28702-992276)

Modifiers never can appear by themselves on a claim form. They must be listed with a proper five-digit CPT code.

Appendix A of the CPT-4 contains a list of available modifiers. Check there first. Then go to the appropriate section of the book to verify that the modifier can be used with the specific CPT code.

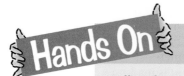

Hands On   USING THE ICD-9-CM   7-1

Follow these steps to use the ICD-9-CM to code patient diagnoses.

1. Choose the main term in the diagnostic statement.
2. Locate the main term in the alphabetic index of Volume 2.
3. Refer to all notes and conventions under the main term.
4. Find the appropriate indented term under the main term.
5. Follow any indicated instructions, such as *see also*.
6. Confirm the code selected from the index by looking it up in Volume 1.
7. Add any fourth or fifth digits provided by Volume 1 as necessary.
8. Assign the code on the claim form.
9. Code the reason for the visit first. Then, code any other conditions that affect the patient's treatment for that visit.
   - Code a chronic condition as long as it applies to the patient's treatment.
   - Don't code a diagnosis that no longer applies.
10. Make sure an ICD-9 code is linked to each service or procedure provided to the patient.
    - For outpatient surgery, code the diagnosis that applies to the procedure.
    - If the postoperative diagnosis differs from the preoperative diagnosis, use the postoperative diagnosis.
11. Identify services for situations other than disease or injury, such as follow-up care, with the appropriate V-code.
    - List the V-code first, followed by the code for the condition.

Hands On

USING THE CPT-4

7-2

Follow these steps to use the CPT-4 book to code services provided to outpatients.

1. Make sure the book you are using is the most current edition of the CPT-4.

2. From the superbill or encounter form, note all the services and procedures provided to the patient during the visit.

3. Find each service or procedure in the index at the back of the CPT book.

4. Find the code the index refers you to for each service or procedure in the appropriate section of the book.

5. Read the description for the code and also any indented descriptions listed under it. Assign the code that most accurately describes the service or procedure.

6. If the service includes an E/M code, verify the code checked on the encounter form by doing the following:
   - Determine whether this is a consultation, a new patient, or an established patient.
   - Verify where the service was performed.
   - Review the documentation to verify the level of service.

7. Verify that each CPT code links correctly with a related diagnostic (ICD-9) code.

8. Check that you have assigned all necessary modifiers and that you haven't coded any bundled procedures separately.

9. Assign the code for each procedure and service and record it on the claim form.

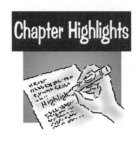

Chapter Highlights

- Diagnostic coding involves using numbers to describe diseases, injuries, and other reasons for seeking medical care.

- Diagnostic coding is linked to reimbursement because it assures that the services and procedures provided by physicians are medically necessary.

- Two volumes of the ICD-9-CM are used in outpatient coding. Volume 1 organizes conditions by type and by body system. Volume 2 organizes them alphabetically by name.

- Procedural coding involves using numbers to describe procedures and other services physicians provide to patients.

- Complete and accurate coding is necessary to ensure proper reimbursement.

- The CPT-4 is used for procedural coding. It is organized by the type of service provided.

- Using the CPT-4 is similar to using the ICD-9-CM because the index in each book is consulted first.

- To ensure accuracy in diagnostic and procedural coding, the most recent version of each book must be used. Office forms also must be kept up to date with the most recent ICD and CPT codes.

Chapter 8

HEALTH INSURANCE AND CLAIMS

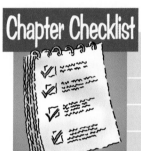

Chapter Checklist

- Describe the differences between group, individual, and government-sponsored health benefit plans

- Explain the difference between Medicare and Medicaid

- Explain how managed care programs work

- Point out similarities and differences between HMOs and PPOs

- Apply third party guidelines

- Apply managed care policies and procedures

- Summarize how to file claims with Medicare, Medicaid, workers' compensation, and private insurance

- Complete insurance claim forms

Perhaps no part of the health care business has changed more in recent years than third-party payment—commonly known as health insurance. Traditional health insurance coverage has largely been replaced by what's called "managed care." Although managed care has simplified the patient's role in paying for services, it has made the job of the administrative medical assistant more complicated. In this chapter, you will learn about the basic types of traditional and managed care health plans. You'll also learn how managed care has affected the process of obtaining third-party payment.

Health Benefit Plans

About 80 percent of Americans are covered by some sort of health benefits plan. This means that most patients who come into the office will have health insurance of one kind or another. These plans can be grouped into three general types.

- group health plans
- individual health benefits policies
- government-sponsored benefits

In addition, group plans and individual policies can be of two types.

- traditional insurance
- managed care

You will read more about traditional insurance and managed care later in the chapter. But no matter the type, payments from health benefits plans provide most of a medical office's income.

As an administrative medical assistant, your work will involve insurance payments. Many of the topics in this book's earlier chapters are related to them, directly or indirectly. Here are some examples.

- collecting insurance information when screening new patients (Chapter 1)
- protecting patient privacy when providing requested medical information (Chapter 2)
- using the Internet to get information about a patient's insurance plan (Chapter 3)
- obtaining the approvals required by some health plans for services and procedures (Chapter 4)
- responding to requests for medical records (Chapter 5)
- performing credit adjustments, issuing refunds, and depositing payments in the office's bank account (Chapter 6)
- coding diagnoses and procedures for filing insurance claims (Chapter 7)

You'll pull together these and other things you've learned to file claims with patients' insurance plans. This is one of the most important jobs in the medical office.

Handling insurance matters effectively also requires that you:

- understand the differences in plans and their requirements so you can complete and file claim forms correctly

- know the special vocabulary involved with health insurance claims
- know how to instruct patients about insurance matters

What you read in this chapter will help you accomplish all three goals.

Though the office's mission is to protect or restore patients' health, it must make money to continue carrying out this mission.

GROUP HEALTH PLANS

A group health plan is sponsored by an organization. Any person who is a member of the organization is eligible to be covered by the plan. If they choose to have this health coverage, they become part of the **group.** Members can usually add their dependents to the group too. **Dependents** generally include the member's spouse and minor children.

Associations and labor unions are among the kinds of organizations that offer these plans. But most group health plans are sponsored by employers. Their workers are eligible for health benefits because of their employment. The employees who decide to be covered are the group in the group plan.

Types of Group Health Plans

You've just read that group plans can be either managed care or traditional insurance. But group health plans can be classified another way too.

- *Insured plans.* These plans can be either managed care or traditional insurance.
- *Self-funded plans.* These plans could be managed care but generally are traditional insurance.

The main difference between insured plans and self-funded plans is in who

---

People's Health   **PPO**

HOSPITAL ADMISSIONS REQUIRE PRIOR APPROVAL

JANE A DOE
BCB9999999 99
GROUP: 285948574449

75.00 EMER ROOM
20.00 OFFICE VISIT

BCBSK RX   1-800-555-1495

BC PLAN: 240 BS PLAN: 740

CUST SERV: 816-555-8346/800-555-2569

Front

To prior authorize all medical or surgical admissions or for
Utilization Management review, call:
816-555-5784 or Toll Free 800-555-5784

If prior approval for a hospital admission is not obtained, the
claim may not be paid. In the event of an emergency admission,
People's Health must be notified within 48 hours.

For Psychiatric and Substance Abuse Services, call:
914-555-5894 or Toll Free 800-555-0948

To locate a participating PPO provider outside of People's Health,
call 800-555-HCARE or visit www.peopleshealth.com.

Health Care Providers must file claims with the LOCAL People's Health
Plan. All other claims must be sent to:
People's Health
PO BOX 90001, Baltimore MD 21201

PBDG

Back

The patient's health plan ID card contains basic information on how to file a claim to a group insurance plan.

manages them and who pays for claims. But in either case, payment from any source but the patient is said to come from a **third-party payer.** The funds received are called third-party reimbursement or **third-party payment.**

Insured Plans. With insured plans, insurance companies charge a fee for benefits. The employer, employee, or both pay this monthly premium.

When a group member receives a health care service, the provider files a claim with the insurance company. If the claim is approved, the company pays the provider. The insurance company's contract with the employer determines which services are covered and which aren't.

Self-Funded Plans. With self-funded plans, the employer itself is the insurer. It hires an insurance company or other company to review claims and make payment from the employer's funds. In this case, the company is only the agent for the plan. Therefore, it's a **third-party administrator** (TPA), not a third-party payer.

Many employers now self-fund their group health plans rather than insure them. This is especially true among large employers that have ample financial resources.

Determining Eligibility

For a group plan to pay an employee's health care expenses, the employee must be eligible for coverage. Eligibility requirements are defined in the policy or plan document. They often include:

- *Work requirement.* The employee must work a minimum number of hours per week.
- *Waiting period.* A stated length of time must pass from the date of employment before health benefits take effect.

To verify a patient's insurance coverage, call the health plan's claims administrator. This phone number usually appears on the patient's health plan ID card.

The employee also must have enrolled in the group. This usually means filling out required forms during an enrollment period. Not all employees will necessarily be members of the group health plan. Group membership is not automatic with employment. Employees must choose to be covered by their employer's health benefits.

The eligibility of a dependent is based on the employee's eligibility. Special requirements may apply to dependent children, however. Usually, they must fit one of these categories.

- unmarried natural or adopted child of the employee
- unmarried stepchild of the employee
- child for whom the employee is legal guardian

In addition, children must be under a maximum age set by the plan. The age limit, however, is usually raised if the child is a full-time student.

INDIVIDUAL HEALTH PLANS

People buy individual health polices from an insurance company. They pay their premiums directly to the insurance company. The insurance company may:

- pay the doctor or hospital directly
- reimburse the person for eligible medical expenses

The process and requirements for filing claims under individual health plans are the same as those for group health plans. Individual policies, however, often offer less coverage than group plans do. For example, the **deductible** for an individual policy may be higher. This is the amount the patient must pay before insurance starts paying.

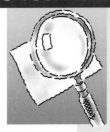

Closer Look HEALTH INSURANCE AND HIPAA

The Health Insurance Portability and Accountability Act of 1996 (HIPAA) brought major changes to the health care and health insurance industries. Here are some ways HIPAA has affected health insurance.

- limited exclusions for preexisting conditions in employer-sponsored health plans
- banned the use of genetic testing information to deny health coverage
- eased confidentiality requirements for providing patient information to insurance companies
- required standards for the electronic transmission of insurance claims
- required standards for attachments to insurance claims
- required diagnostic and procedural coding to be standardized
- strengthened protections against fraud and abuse in insurance billing

An individual policy also may have a provision that denies or limits benefits for certain **preexisting conditions.** These are injuries or illnesses the patient had before the policy took effect. Sometimes, these conditions are not covered even if the patient was not being treated for them at the time.

Preexisting conditions generally won't apply to most patients covered by group health plans. That's because the Health Insurance Portability and Accountability Act of 1996 (HIPAA) severely limited this exclusion in employer-sponsored plans.

GOVERNMENT HEALTH PLANS

Government-sponsored health benefit programs are funded and operated by the federal government and the individual states. These programs are designed to provide health benefits for the elderly, the poor, and others who might not be able to get benefits on their own. The main government programs are:

- Medicare
- Medicaid
- TRICARE
- CHAMPVA

Medicare

Congress created Medicare in the 1960s as a health benefits plan for persons age 65 and over. At the time, only about half of elderly Americans had health insurance coverage.

All persons who are entitled to receive Social Security retirement benefits become eligible for Medicare when they reach age 65. This is true even if they don't retire. But as long as they are covered by an employer's group health plan, that plan is the primary coverage and Medicare is secondary.

In the 1970s, Congress expanded the Medicare program to cover other groups who had difficulty obtaining health insurance. These groups include:

- disabled persons who cannot work and are receiving Social Security disability benefits; they must receive these benefits for 24 months before they are eligible for Medicare.
- persons suffering from end-stage renal disease; these are persons whose kidneys have failed permanently and who are receiving dialysis.

In recent years, Congress changed Medicare again, to create more choices for coverage. The early Medicare program (now called *Original Medicare*) consisted of two parts.

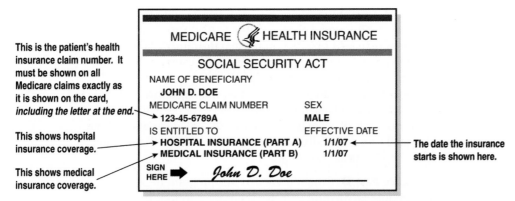

This is the patient's health insurance claim number. It must be shown on all Medicare claims exactly as it is shown on the card, *including the letter at the end.*

This shows hospital insurance coverage.

This shows medical insurance coverage.

The date the insurance starts is shown here.

A patient's Medicare ID card shows whether the patient has Part B coverage for physician's services. It also provides the patient's claim number and Medicare's toll-free information number.

- Medicare Part A covers hospital expenses.
- Medicare Part B pays for physicians' services.

Eligible persons still may enroll in Original Medicare, or they may choose what's called Medicare Advantage instead.

Medicare Part A. Everyone enrolled in Original Medicare is covered by Part A. There's no monthly charge for this coverage, although the plan has deductibles and **coinsurance.** Coinsurance is money a patient must pay as his share of the cost of treatment. Since Part A is a hospital plan, you probably won't be dealing with it much in an outpatient medical office.

Medicare Part B. Medicare Part B is optional. Patients who have this coverage pay a monthly fee deducted from their Social Security checks.

Part B pays physicians' fees for both inpatient and outpatient care. It also pays for a number of other services. Here are some examples.

- diagnostic testing
- certain immunizations such as influenza and pneumonia
- specific screening tests such as PSA, mammograms, Pap smears, bone density testing, and colorectal screening
- medical equipment such as canes, crutches, walkers, commodes, and chairs

All Part B charges are subject to deductibles and coinsurance. A number of other requirements also apply. You'll learn about them later, when you read about filing claims with Medicare and private insurance.

Medicare Advantage. Medicare Advantage used to be called Medicare + Choice and Medicare Part C. This program offers a variety of managed care and traditional insurance plans through private insurance companies. Patients may choose one of them as an option to Original Medicare.

These plans operate much like other managed care and traditional insurance plans. But their benefits have been adjusted to meet the needs of older patients. Most of the information about managed care and traditional insurance that you will read later applies to Medicare Advantage too.

Medicare Part D. Congress created this program in 2003 to help people on Medicare pay for their prescription drugs. The program began in January 2006. Like Medicare Part B, it's voluntary. People must choose to have this coverage.

Medicare Part D is like Part B in some other ways too.

- Recipients must pay a monthly fee for this plan.
- Deductibles and co-payments apply to the coverage.

A **co-payment** is a small payment a patient must make toward his bill. Unlike coinsurance, it's usually a fixed amount—such as $10 for a prescription or an office visit.

People enrolled in Medicare Advantage plans may already have better drug benefits than those offered by Part D. Like Medicare Advantage, the Medicare Part D plans are offered through private companies.

MEDIGAP

Medigap is the name given to policies that private companies sell to fill the gaps in Original Medicare. These polices are voluntary and cost the patient an additional monthly fee. They pay for things Medicare Parts A and B do not. For example, a Medigap policy may pay the following gaps in Part B coverage:

- the annual deductible
- coinsurance for physicians' services
- an annual physical examination
- other services, treatments, and supplies not covered by Medicare

Medicare generally will bill Medigap for you when it pays your claim. You don't need to file a separate claim with the patient's Medigap insurance company. Just be sure to check on the claim to make sure the Medigap policy was filed and paid for.

Medicaid

Many poor people receive their health care through Medicaid. The federal government provides funds to the states to help cover Medicaid costs. Each state is required to provide a Medicaid program.

Medicaid Eligibility. A patient's eligibility for Medicaid is often based on his eligibility for other state programs, such as welfare assistance. So eligibility can vary from state to state. But here are some examples of people who probably will qualify for Medicaid.

- minor children whose family's income is under the poverty level; this figure is set by the federal government and depends on family size.

- persons who receive Aid to Families with Dependent Children (AFDC); this is a program for low-income parents with children under age 18.

- persons who receive Supplemental Security Income (SSI); this is a program for people whose disabilities keep them from working but who aren't eligible for Social Security disability.

Medicaid Coverage. The federal government sets Medicaid's minimum coverage. But states can provide coverage beyond the minimum. Therefore, like eligibility for Medicaid, benefits vary from state to state. All states provide at least these coverages:

- inpatient hospital care

- outpatient treatment and services

- diagnostic services

- family planning

- skilled nursing facilities

- diagnostic screenings for children

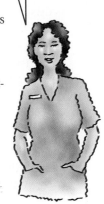

Medicaid is always secondary to Medicare or private insurance. Bill Medicaid only after these sources have paid.

Working with Medicaid. Because Medicaid payments are low, not all doctors take part in Medicaid. If your office accepts Medicaid patients, you'll need to be familiar with the Medicaid program in your state.

Most states require you to get approval from Medicaid before you provide treatment. Here are some examples of state regulations.

- Some states have adopted a managed care approach to their Medicaid programs. Patients are assigned to a primary care physician (PCP) who provides basic care. The PCP then refers the patient to other physicians as needed.

Closer Look · MEDICAID ID CARDS

Medicaid ID cards can vary from state to state.

- In some states, Medicaid patients receive a new ID card each month. Make a photocopy of this card for the patient's record on the first visit of the month.
- Other states issue a more permanent ID card. You verify coverage by swiping this card through a special machine that's like a credit card reader. You should verify coverage for patients with this type of card each time they come into the office.

If you refer a Medicaid patient to another provider, first be sure that provider accepts Medicaid. The law requires providers to accept Medicaid payment as payment in full. They can't bill patients unless it's for something Medicaid doesn't cover.

TRICARE and CHAMPVA

TRICARE used to be known as CHAMPUS. This government program is run by the U.S. Department of Defense. It provides health benefits for:

- dependents of active duty military personnel
- dependents of military personnel who died while on active duty
- retired military personnel and their dependents

The TRICARE system provides health care through civilian hospitals and clinics. The original CHAMPUS was like traditional insurance. In the 1990s, Congress acted to control its costs by adding two managed care options. These three choices form the TRICARE program.

- *TRICARE Standard.* This is the old CHAMPUS plan. Patients have their choice of providers and pay yearly deductibles and coinsurance.
- *TRICARE Extra.* This option is like TRICARE Standard except that patients must obtain their care from an approved list of providers. Patient payments are lower for those who choose this plan.
- *TRICARE Prime.* Patients are assigned a primary case manager (PCM) who must approve all care before it is provided.

The PCM is named on the patient's TRICARE Prime ID card. Patients pay no deductibles with this option.

CHAMPVA. CHAMPVA stands for the Civilian Health and Medical Program of the Veterans Administration. It covers dependents of two types of military veterans. These are:

- dependents of veterans who have total and permanent service-connected disabilities
- dependents of veterans who died from service-connected disabilities

CHAMPVA patients can choose their own civilian physician. This allows them the same benefits as a traditional insurance program.

Traditional Health Insurance

You have learned that health benefits can come from group plans, individual policies, and government-sponsored plans. You've also seen that some plans can be managed care plans and others can be traditional insurance.

Billing and Traditional Insurance

Traditional insurance plans often are called fee-for-service plans. Here's how they work.

1. The patient goes to a provider of her choice.
2. The provider submits bills (claims) for treating the patient to the patient's insurance company.
3. The company pays the bills according to the terms of the policy or plan, minus any deductibles or patient coinsurance.
4. The provider credits the insurance payment to the patient's account.
5. The provider bills any deductibles and coinsurance to the patient.

The provider also may bill the patient for any other amounts not paid by insurance. For example, the insurance company's maximum allowable payment for a service may be less than the provider's fee. In some cases, the provider can require the patient to pay the difference. Also, an insurance plan may not cover certain equipment or supplies.

Types of Traditional Insurance

Most traditional insurance plans provide the following kinds of coverage.

- Basic medical benefits pay all or part of a physician's charges for nonsurgical services. These include office, hospital, and home visits as well as most lab tests and x-rays. Many plans don't pay for routine physical examinations, however. To be paid, the exam must be related to a specific patient complaint.

- Hospitalization coverage pays all or part of the costs for a patient's hospital room, food, and health care services that don't involve a physician. It also pays for use of hospital facilities, such as an operating room.

- Surgical coverage pays all or part of a surgeon's fees. The surgery can take place in the hospital or the physician's office. If the procedure requires anesthesia, this is paid by the surgical benefits as well.

- Major medical coverage pays for very large bills that can result from a long or extremely serious illness. This coverage usually takes effect when benefits under the plan's other coverages have been exhausted.

Deductibles and coinsurance usually apply to most of these coverages. If major medical coverage is in effect, however, the patient may have already paid his maximum required amount.

Managed Care

Over the past 30 years, health care costs have grown at about twice the rate of inflation. As a result, private insurers have developed systems to keep costs down by managing health care. Today, managed care plans are more common than traditional health insurance. Even the government has followed this trend. It offers managed care plans such as Medicare Advantage, TRICARE Extra, and TRICARE Prime.

In traditional insurance systems, the patient has a contractual relationship with the provider. (You read about contracts and the physician-patient relationship in Chapter 2.) The provider decides what care is needed and bills the patient's health plan. The plan pays the provider. The insurer has no other relationship with the provider.

In managed care systems, the insurer has a contractual relationship with the provider. The contract usually sets the price that will be charged for each service. It also sets the conditions under which the service will be covered.

MANAGING COSTS

Managed care plans control costs in several ways.

- *Networks.* A network is a group of physicians, hospitals, pharmacies, and others who have agreed to provide services to patients in a health plan at a set price. The patient is required to use network providers to receive full coverage. If he goes outside the network for care, his coverage is reduced greatly.

- *Precertification.* Most insurance plans require that certain procedures are precertified before the patient can receive the treatment. These usually include hospitalization and other procedures except in emergencies. The goal is to provide services in the most cost-effective way. For example, surgeries for which patients were once hospitalized are now performed in outpatient settings. Precertification is sometimes called utilization management (UM) or utilization review (UR).

> Precertifications and approvals are very important. A managed care plan can deny payment if there was no approval or precertification, and you can't bill the patient instead.

- *Approved referrals.* Many managed care plans will not pay for treatment by specialists unless the patient is referred by his primary care physician, or PCP. Some plans require preapproval by the plan administrator as well. The goal is to ensure that a specialist's services are medically necessary.

- *Assignment of benefits.* A network provider may not bill the patient for any amounts not paid by the plan, except for co-payments, coinsurance, and deductibles. This is managed care's way of enforcing precertification and approval requirements.

Managing Managed Care

Most physicians have contracts with more than one managed care program. It's likely that your office will be part of several managed care networks. Each of these plans will have its own reimbursement schedule and set of requirements. To bring the most reimbursement possible into the office, you'll need to consider the requirements of each patient's program.

Knowing UM or precertification requirements is extremely important. They may apply only to inpatient services or to a variety of outpatient and office services as well. Check the patient's ID card carefully for these details.

It's also important to be familiar with the providers in each network. The physician, hospital, or other provider you refer one patient to might not be in another patient's network. By calling the UM number to check, you can avoid the financial penalties that can result from making a mistake.

Use the Hands On procedure on page 289 as a general guide to following the policies and procedures of managed care plans.

HEALTH MAINTENANCE ORGANIZATIONS

Unlike traditional insurance plans, a health maintenance organization (HMO) provides services rather than just paying for them. Thus an HMO is both an insurer and a provider.

HMO policies are written differently than traditional insurance policies. An HMO policy lists the services the insured is entitled to receive. It also lists the providers who will perform those services.

HMOs deliver services to their members in two ways.

- using their own staff of physicians and hospitals

- contracting with physicians and hospitals for the services

When a patient belongs to an HMO, she's not responsible for her bill. Instead, the HMO is. Many HMOs require the patient to make a small co-payment—such as $10 per physician office visit. But deductibles and coinsurance generally do not apply.

You should collect an HMO member's co-payment at the time of the visit. For this reason, an HMO patient will never see a bill from your

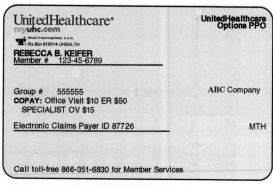

UnitedHealthcare®
myuhc.com
PAID Prescriptions, L.L.C.
Rx Bin 610014 UHEALTH
UnitedHealthcare Options PPO

REBECCA B. KEIFER
Member #   123-45-6789

Group #   555555
COPAY: Office Visit $10 ER $50
   SPECIALIST OV $15

ABC Company

Electronic Claims Payer ID 87726

MTH

Call toll-free 866-351-6830 for Member Services

This card does not prove membership nor guarantee coverage. For verification of benefits, please call Member Services.

IMPORTANT MEMBER INFORMATION
For authorization of health care services specific to your plan, you must call the number on the front of this card prior to the service to receive the highest level of benefits (see your benefit description for details). In emergencies, call Member Services within 48 hours.

Claim Address: PO BOX 740800, Atlanta, GA 30374-0800

United HealthCare Insurance Company   Issued:01/04/03

Here's a sample ID card for a managed care plan.

Closer Look

TYPES OF HMOs

Some HMOs pay providers a fee for each service. This amount is determined by the HMO's fee schedule. Often, the HMO will withhold part of each payment until the end of the year. Then, if the HMO's total medical expense is within budget, it will pay the withheld amounts to the physician.

Other HMOs are called capitated HMOs because they pay by **capitation.** This means they pay the provider a single, set amount for each patient's care. The amount is the same, no matter how much or how little care is required. Most capitated HMOs still require physicians to submit claim forms. This lets them track the services each physician is providing.

Capitation and the withholding of fees are both ways by which HMOs encourage physicians to be cost-conscious in caring for patients.

office. You must understand the type of relationship your office has with an HMO, however, before you can know what other reimbursement to expect.

Gatekeepers

Gatekeeper provisions are common in HMOs. Other managed care organizations sometimes have gatekeepers as well.

A **gatekeeper** is a primary care physician (PCP). Plans that use gatekeepers require each member to choose a PCP from lists of providers. The member must go to her PCP for all care except for emergencies. The PCP treats the patient or, if necessary, refers her to another provider. In many cases, the PCP also must obtain the plan's approval for the referral.

One purpose of gatekeepers is to reduce the use and cost of specialists. Without the gatekeeper requirement, a patient might see a specialist first. This would result in a costly fee, when the condition might have been treated at lower cost by the PCP. The gatekeeper approach also encourages patients to develop a strong relationship with one physician, who is then in a good position to manage their care.

PREFERRED PROVIDER ORGANIZATIONS

A preferred provider organization (PPO) is a network of physicians, hospitals, and other providers that contracts with one or more health plans. The PPO's members agree to accept less than their normal charges and to follow the plan's requirements for providing services.

Unlike an HMO, patients in a health plan with a PPO can go to any provider they wish. The plan generally offers two levels of service, called *in-network* and *out-of-network*.

- If the provider is in-network (called a **participating provider**), the plan's benefits are greater.
- If the provider is out-of-network (called a nonparticipating provider), the patient must pay more.

The table below illustrates this point.

Although the PPO system gives patients free choice, they have a strong financial incentive to see in-network providers. The health plan's reward when they do this is the reduced fees in-network providers charge for their services.

A Health Plan with a PPO

Benefit	In-Network	Out-of-Network
Yearly patient deductible	$100	$300
Patient coinsurance	10%	30%
Routine care benefit	$200 per year	0
Mental health benefit	80% of charges	50% of charges
Office visit—patient share	$10 co-pay; no deductible	70% of charges

PPOs and You

As an administrative medical assistant, you'll need to know about each PPO to which your office belongs. At the very least, your knowledge must include:

- familiarity with the PPO's fee schedule as it applies to the services your office provides
- knowledge of the procedures the PPO's contract with the patient's health plan requires the office to follow
- awareness of the administrative support the physician's contract with the PPO requires the office to provide

Most participating providers have agreed to certain conditions in their relationship with a PPO's patients. Here are the most common of these requirements.

- Comply with all plan procedures for precertifications and referrals.
- Collect the co-pay amount at the time of service.
- Accept assignment of benefits from the patient.
- File all claims for the patient.
- Accept the plan's reimbursement as payment in full (after any deductibles and coinsurance).
- Agree not to bill the patient for any difference between the physician's usual charge and the PPO's negotiated fee for the service.

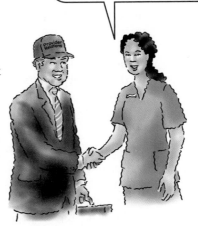

Most PPOs have provider relations representatives who'll answer your questions and clarify the PPO's requirements and procedures.

Filing Claims

Many pieces of information are needed for claims processing. A patient's health plan cannot process a claim if you've provided incomplete or inaccurate information. Claims that don't follow a plan's required procedures also must be returned for resubmission. The provider will have to wait longer for payment as a result. This makes submitting accurate claims a critical part of your administrative responsibilities. The Hands On procedure on page 290 provides guidelines to make your claims filing efficient.

At the same time, the patients seen in the office may have coverage from a large number of health plans. Some of these plans may be PPOs or HMOs; others may be traditional insurance. Your challenge will be to keep track of the coverage—and not to take benefits for granted or guess when you're not sure.

The patient's ID card is your basic resource for processing insurance. This card contains information that's essential to the accurate filing of claims.

- the name of the plan that provides the patient's coverage
- the patient's plan ID number and group number if it's group coverage
- phone numbers for questions about benefits, coverages, and approval requirements
- directions on where to file claims

Keep a copy of the patient's ID card in the patient's file. Update it at least yearly. Also verify the information at each visit, since the patient's employment and eligibility may change.

Coordination of Benefits

It's not uncommon for a patient to be eligible for benefits from more than one health plan. For example, a patient may be covered under her employer's plan and also as a dependent on her spouse's group plan. The plan that pays first—the primary plan—is the plan provided by the patient's employer. The spouse's group plan is secondary. It will consider any amounts up to the allowable limit for the policy not paid by the primary insurance. This is called **coordination of benefits.**

THE BIRTHDAY RULE

Dependent children may be covered on the plans of both parents. When this happens, the primary plan is usually the plan of the parent whose birthday occurs first during the year (not necessarily the oldest parent). This is known as the **birthday rule.**

Consider this example of a married couple:

- Brad's birthday is December 20, 1963.
- Maria's birthday is October 11, 1965

Whose insurance would be primary? It would be Maria because the month and day of her birthday come before Brad's. It doesn't matter that Brad is the older of the two.

If the parents are divorced or legally separated, the primary plan is usually the plan of the parent who has custody. In some instances, however, a court order or the divorce decree may make the other parent's plan primary.

> Remember, when using the birthday rule, it's the date that matters, not the age.

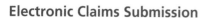

Electronic Claims Submission

Once you've established the primary plan, the next step is to prepare the claim for filing. The patient's insurance card should contain information on how and where to file. The CMS-1500 is the standard form for filing claims. It is accepted by almost all claims administrators, including Medicare, Medicaid, TRICARE, and CHAMPVA.

HIPAA requires that all claims, with very few exceptions, be filed electronically—that is, by computer. Several regional and national clearinghouses receive these claims and electronically direct them to the proper claims administrators. This system allows you to send all claims to one place instead of filing each one separately with many different claims administrators.

The system also requires that all fields on the electronic claim form be completed and in the required format. The Hands On procedure on page 291 provides you with line-by-line guidance for doing this.

The system will reject any claims that don't meet the requirements of the patient's health plan. If this happens, they usually must be submitted by mail. Claims that are very complicated, or those with many attachments such as lab results or x-rays, also should be submitted to the plan's claims administrator on paper.

Assignment of Benefits

Assignment of benefits is a service your office may provide. This allows the health plan to pay the office directly. The

Closer Look

DENIED CLAIMS: TAKING CORRECTIVE ACTION

Denied claims can lead to lengthy delays in payment to the physician. Here are the most frequent reasons for denial of a claim and actions you should take to address them.

- *The patient cannot be identified as a covered person.* Confirm that the coverage information on file is correct, including the health plan's name, policy or group number, and the patient's Social Security number.

- *Coding is not appropriate for the services provided.* Review provided services and recode as necessary.

- *The patient is no longer covered by the plan.* Bill the patient for the charges. The patient may produce evidence of new coverage.

- *The data are incomplete.* Complete the required data and resubmit the claim.

- *The services are not covered by the plan.* Bill the patient for the services unless there's a basis for an appeal.

office typically delays billing the patient until the insurance claim is paid. The patient is then billed for any remaining charges if the office's contract with the patient's health plan allows it.

Most managed care plans require participating providers to accept assignment of benefits. Here's what you'll need to do.

- Have the patient sign a form assigning the insurance benefits to the office.
- Keep this signature on file so the patient will not have to sign this section on the claim form each time.
- Finally, enter *signature on file* on the patient's signature line when you file the claim.

Some physicians don't accept assignment for patients who have traditional insurance. If this applies to your office, the patient will be responsible for paying the charges and for filing the claim with his health plan himself. The plan would send the check to the patient.

Balance Billing. Most managed care plans also prohibit **balance billing.** This is the practice of billing the patient for the difference between the physician's usual charge and the health plan's allowable charge.

Balance billing isn't done in managed care because the plan's contract with its in-network providers requires that the allowable charge be accepted as full payment. For other types of private insurance, however, you may bill the patient for the difference.

Explanation of Benefits

When a claims administrator settles a claim, it sends an **explanation of benefits** (EOB) to both the patient and the provider. The EOB tells about the payment (if any) the plan made. It also includes information about deductible amounts and coinsurance as they apply to the claim. The sample EOB on page 287 explains this sometimes confusing form in detail.

Some EOBs include information for several claims for several patients the plan has processed during a stated period. You may be responsible for checking EOBs to make sure all payments are for the correct procedures and amounts. These payments will be credited to the patients' accounts and any deductibles and coinsurance billed to the patient. (You read about billing and patients' accounts in Chapter 5.)

Explanation of Benefits

Employee Name: Joe Doe
SSN: 555-55-5555   1
Group No. 55555
Patient Name: Joe Doe

Date of Service: 6-15-2004
Provider: Dr. Jones
Provider TIN: 35-5555555

Date of Service 2	Comment Code 3	Amount of Charge 4	Amount Allowed 5	At 6	Amount Paid 7
6-15-2007	57	87.00	82.00	80%	65.60
			Total 8		65.60
			Less Deductible 9		25.00
			Amount Paid 10		40.60

Payable to: Dr. Jones
              Address

Comment Code:
57 - The amount charged exceeds Usual and Customary

Reading the EOB (Explanation of Benefits)

Although each health plan has its own EOB form, this sample shows an EOB's key information.

1. The top information includes the name and Social Security number of the policyholder, plus the patient's name. That name will be different if the patient is a dependent of the insured.

2. This column shows the specific date each service included on the claim was provided.

3. This column is used to explain adjustments to the payment for each service. The code numbers refer to comments at the bottom of the page. In this case, the physician's charge (4) exceeded the payment this plan allows for the service (5). Unless the physician is required to accept the plan's amount as full payment, the patient can be billed for this difference.

4. This is the charge the physician submitted to the patient's health plan.

5. This is the maximum amount the plan will pay for this service.

6. The plan has paid 80 percent of its allowed amount. The other 20 percent is coinsurance that should be billed to the patient.

7. This is the plan's 80-percent share of its allowable amount for this service, after coinsurance.

8. This is the total of the amount in column 7.

9. Any unpaid amount remaining in the patient's annual deductible is subtracted from what the plan will pay.

10. This is the amount actually paid by the plan. Although each health plan has its own EOB form, this sample shows an EOB's key information.

FILING WORKERS' COMPENSATION CLAIMS

Employees in every state are covered by a workers' compensation program. This program is operated by the state or by a TPA the state hires to run the plan. The plan's benefits cover medical expenses resulting from work-related illnesses or injuries.

If you bill the patient's health plan for services related to a work-related condition, the plan will return your claim with instructions to file it with the workers' compensation claims administrator.

When your office treats patients for injuries, always inquire if the injury is work-related. Also be aware that some illnesses can be work-related too. It's important to know this before services are provided so you can account and file for the charges correctly.

FILING CLAIMS AND MEDICARE

If your office accepts Medicare, you must file all Medicare claims for the patient. Medicare providers cannot require patients to file their own claims. All physicians who accept Medicare must file the claims for payment.

> Know your state's requirements for treating patients under workers' compensation. You can get this information from your state's workers' compensation office or its claims administrator.

Most physicians are participating providers (PAR providers) with Medicare. To be PAR providers, they must agree to Medicare's fee schedule. They submit the bill to Medicare and get payment in return. The payment will be for 80 percent of the Medicare-approved amount for the service. The remaining 20 percent is patient coinsurance.

PAR providers can bill a Medicare patient for the coinsurance and also for any deductible amount. But balance billing is not allowed. This makes PAR providers much like members of a PPO. They must accept the insurer's approved fee as payment in full.

Physicians who aren't PAR providers also must file the patient's claim. But Medicare will send the payment to the patient instead. This means non-PAR providers must collect both Medicare's share and the coinsurance from the patient. However, non-PAR providers are permitted to balance bill patients for charges that exceed what Medicare allows.

Some non-PAR providers ask patients to make part or full payment at the time of the service. This can be a financial hardship for the patient, especially until the patient is reimbursed by Medicare.

Crossover Claims. Medicare patients whose financial hardship is great may be excused from paying the 20 percent coinsurance. In some cases, such patients also may be eligible for Medicaid. This is referred to as a **crossover claim** because the unpaid amount of the Medicare claim crosses over automatically to Medicaid.

When a patient is covered by both Medicare and Medicaid, bill Medicare first. Medicare is always primary and Medicaid is secondary. Always ask Medicare patients if they have any other coverage. Many who are not eligible for Medicaid may have Medigap insurance.

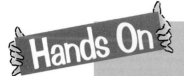

OBTAINING PREAPPROVALS FROM MANAGED CARE PLANS

8-1

Follow these steps before sending patients covered by managed care plans to other providers for referrals, consultations, or expensive tests.

1. Gather the patient's chart and the office's copy of the patient's health plan ID card.

2. Locate the patient's ID number and the plan's information phone number on the ID card. (Note that some cards may contain a special phone number for authorizations.)

3. Obtain the patient's diagnosis from the chart.

4. Determine the provider to which the physician wants the patient sent.

5. Check to be sure the provider is on the plan's list of approved providers.
   - Many plans make approved provider information available online.
   - The plan's information handbook is another source of approved provider information.

6. Call the plan with the above information and verify the following:
   - that an approval is necessary
   - that the provider is still an approved provider with the plan

7. Get an authorization code if approval is necessary and document it in the patient's chart.
   - If approval is not necessary, document that information in the patient's chart.
   - Include in all documentation the date, time, and name of the person you spoke with at the plan.

8. Fax a copy of the authorization, if required, to the provider to whom the patient is being sent.

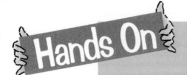

FOLLOWING THIRD PARTY GUIDELINES WHEN FILING CLAIMS

8-2

Here's a checklist of things to remember when filing a claim with any third-party payer or claims administrator. Following these tips will increase the office's income and lessen the chances of rejected claims or delayed payments.

1. Determine whether the plan's coverage is primary or secondary and file charges accordingly.

2. Check that the patient's personal information on the claim form is accurate and complete.

3. Check that the identifying information about the insurance plan, group number, insured's ID number, and so on is accurate and complete.

4. Make sure ICD and CPT coding are accurate and complete. Each CPT code being billed should be supported by a specific ICD code.

5. Determine whether the health plan accepts or requires assignment of benefits. If so, make sure the insured's signature is provided on the claim form or is on file in the office.

6. Determine if the plan requires coinsurance, co-payments, or deductibles from the insured. If so, make sure these are billed if appropriate.

7. Be aware of any health plan regulations requiring approval of referrals and certain procedures.
   - In some cases, these may require only a prescription from the physician.
   - In other cases, an authorization code may be needed.
   - Call the plan's claims administrator if there's any doubt.

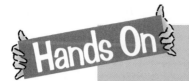

PREPARING A CMS-1500 FOR SUBMISSION

8-3

Follow these steps in completing a CMS-1500. Each number in this procedure refers to the area with the same number on the form.

1. Check off where the claim is being submitted.

1a. Enter the ID number of the insured.
   - This may not be the patient's ID number.
   - Entering the patient's number here instead of the insured's number will cause the claim to be rejected.
   - If the patient is covered by more than one policy, the primary policyholder's number goes here.

2. Enter the patient's name in the correct order—last, first, middle initial.

3. Provide the patient's date of birth. There should be eight digits (mmddyyyy).

4. Enter the name of the insured. Again, make sure this is the insured's name, if the insured is not the patient.

5. Provide the patient's address.

6. Indicate the patient's relationship to the insured.

7. Enter the insured's address.

8. Indicate the patient's status. Be sure to check a box in both areas.

9. If the patient is covered by more than one person's plan, enter the name of the secondary insurance policyholder on this line.
   - A child may be covered on the insurance plan of each parent.
   - An adult may be covered on an employer's plan and on a spouse's employer plan as well.

9a. Provide the secondary insured's policy or group number.

9b. Indicate the secondary insured's date of birth and gender.

9c. Enter the secondary insured's employer or school name.

9d. Provide the name of the secondary insured's insurance plan.

10. Check the appropriate boxes concerning the reason for the patient's condition.

11. Provide the group number of the primary insured's policy.

11a. Indicate the primary insured's date of birth and gender.

(continued)

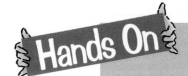

PREPARING A CMS-1500 FOR SUBMISSION (*continued*)

8-3

11b. Enter the primary insured's employer or school name.

11c. Provide the name of the primary insured's insurance plan.

11d. Indicate whether there is secondary insurance. If so, fill out section 9 as noted above.

12. The patient's signature on this line authorizes your office to receive payment directly from the health plan.
    - It also allows the release of medical information to the plan to process the claim.
    - If you have the patient's signature on file in the office, you may enter "signature on file" on this line.

13. If the insured is other than the patient, the insured's signature is needed here to assign benefits to the office.

14. Place the date the current illness or injury began here. This may *not* be the date of treatment or service.

15. If the patient has had this condition before, enter the date of the first occurrence.

16. If the patient is unable to work, enter the dates of disability.

17. If the patient has been referred to the office, provide the name of the referring physician.

17a. Enter the EIN of the referring physician.

18. If the patient has been hospitalized for this condition, enter the dates of hospital admission and discharge.

20. If charges were incurred by an outside lab, check *yes* and enter the amount of the charges. Otherwise, check *no*.

21. Enter up to four ICD-9 codes in this box. List the primary diagnosis code on line 1.

22. This is required only for a replacement claim to Medicaid.

23. If a service being billed required preapproval by the health plan, enter the approval number here.

24a. Enter the dates of service.

24b–d. Using CPT or HCPCS codes, enter the place and type of service and the procedures performed.

24e. Use this box to connect each procedure with the appropriate line in box 21.

24f. Enter the charge for each listed service or procedure.

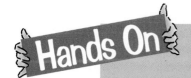

**PREPARING A CMS-1500
FOR SUBMISSION** (*continued*)

8-3

24g. This is the number of visits, units of supplies, etc. Most often the number entered here will be 1.

24h–k. These are special-use boxes for certain kinds of claims.

25. Enter the physician's tax ID number and indicate if it is a Social Security number or an employer identification number.

26. If your office has assigned an account number to the patient, enter it here.

27. Indicate whether your office accepts assignment of benefits.

28. Enter the total charges for the service listed in box 24.

29. Indicate any amounts already paid by the patient.
    • If the patient owes coinsurance or deductibles but has not paid them, leave this line blank.

30. Enter the balance due.

31. The physician's signature may be typed, stamped, or written in this box. The date it is "signed" also must be provided.

32. If the service was provided outside the office, enter the address where the service was provided.

33. Enter your office's name, address, and phone number. If benefits have been assigned, payment will be sent to this address.

PLEASE
DO NOT
STAPLE
IN THIS
AREA

HEALTH INSURANCE CLAIM FORM

| | PICA | | | | | | | PICA | | |

CARRIER

1. MEDICARE   MEDICAID   CHAMPUS   CHAMPVA   GROUP HEALTH PLAN   FECA BLK LUNG   OTHER   1a. INSURED'S I.D. NUMBER   (FOR PROGRAM IN ITEM 1)

☐ (Medicare #) ☐ (Medicaid #) ☐ (Sponsor's SSN) ☐ (VA File #) ☐ (SSN or ID) ☐ (SSN) ☐ (ID)

2. PATIENT'S NAME (Last Name, First Name, Middle Initial)

3. PATIENT'S BIRTH DATE MM DD YY   SEX M ☐ F ☐

4. INSURED'S NAME (Last Name, First Name, Middle Initial)

5. PATIENT'S ADDRESS (No., Street)

6. PATIENT RELATIONSHIP TO INSURED Self ☐ Spouse ☐ Child ☐ Other ☐

7. INSURED'S ADDRESS (No., Street)

CITY   STATE

8. PATIENT STATUS Single ☐ Married ☐ Other ☐ Employed ☐ Full-Time Student ☐ Part-Time Student ☐

CITY   STATE

ZIP CODE   TELEPHONE (Include Area Code) (   )

ZIP CODE   TELEPHONE (INCLUDE AREA CODE) (   )

9. OTHER INSURED'S NAME (Last Name, First Name, Middle Initial)

10. IS PATIENT'S CONDITION RELATED TO:

11. INSURED'S POLICY GROUP OR FECA NUMBER

a. OTHER INSURED'S POLICY OR GROUP NUMBER

a. EMPLOYMENT? (CURRENT OR PREVIOUS) ☐ YES ☐ NO

a. INSURED'S DATE OF BIRTH MM DD YY   SEX M ☐ F ☐

b. OTHER INSURED'S DATE OF BIRTH MM DD YY   SEX M ☐ F ☐

b. AUTO ACCIDENT? PLACE (State) ☐ YES ☐ NO

b. EMPLOYER'S NAME OR SCHOOL NAME

c. EMPLOYER'S NAME OR SCHOOL NAME

c. OTHER ACCIDENT? ☐ YES ☐ NO

c. INSURANCE PLAN NAME OR PROGRAM NAME

d. INSURANCE PLAN NAME OR PROGRAM NAME

10d. RESERVED FOR LOCAL USE

d. IS THERE ANOTHER HEALTH BENEFIT PLAN? ☐ YES ☐ NO *If yes,* return to and complete item 9 a-d.

PATIENT AND INSURED INFORMATION

READ BACK OF FORM BEFORE COMPLETING & SIGNING THIS FORM.
12. PATIENT'S OR AUTHORIZED PERSON'S SIGNATURE I authorize the release of any medical or other information necessary to process this claim. I also request payment of government benefits either to myself or to the party who accepts assignment below.

SIGNED _____ DATE _____

13. INSURED'S OR AUTHORIZED PERSON'S SIGNATURE I authorize payment of medical benefits to the undersigned physician or supplier for services described below.

SIGNED _____

14. DATE OF CURRENT: ILLNESS (First symptom) OR MM DD YY   INJURY (Accident) OR PREGNANCY(LMP)

15. IF PATIENT HAS HAD SAME OR SIMILAR ILLNESS. GIVE FIRST DATE MM DD YY

16. DATES PATIENT UNABLE TO WORK IN CURRENT OCCUPATION MM DD YY FROM   TO MM DD YY

17. NAME OF REFERRING PHYSICIAN OR OTHER SOURCE

17a. I.D. NUMBER OF REFERRING PHYSICIAN

18. HOSPITALIZATION DATES RELATED TO CURRENT SERVICES MM DD YY FROM   TO MM DD YY

19. RESERVED FOR LOCAL USE

20. OUTSIDE LAB? ☐ YES ☐ NO $ CHARGES

21. DIAGNOSIS OR NATURE OF ILLNESS OR INJURY. (RELATE ITEMS 1,2,3 OR 4 TO ITEM 24E BY LINE)

1. ⌊___⌋ . ⌊___⌋   3. ⌊___⌋ . ⌊___⌋
2. ⌊___⌋ . ⌊___⌋   4. ⌊___⌋ . ⌊___⌋

22. MEDICAID RESUBMISSION CODE   ORIGINAL REF. NO.

23. PRIOR AUTHORIZATION NUMBER

24. A DATE(S) OF SERVICE From To MM DD YY MM DD YY	B Place of Service	C Type of Service	D PROCEDURES, SERVICES, OR SUPPLIES (Explain Unusual Circumstances) CPT/HCPCS MODIFIER	E DIAGNOSIS CODE	F $ CHARGES	G DAYS OR UNITS	H EPSDT Family Plan	I EMG	J COB	K RESERVED FOR LOCAL USE
1										
2										
3										
4										
5										
6										

PHYSICIAN OR SUPPLIER INFORMATION

25. FEDERAL TAX I.D. NUMBER   SSN EIN ☐ ☐

26. PATIENT'S ACCOUNT NO.

27. ACCEPT ASSIGNMENT? (For govt. claims, see back) ☐ YES ☐ NO

28. TOTAL CHARGE $

29. AMOUNT PAID $

30. BALANCE DUE $

31. SIGNATURE OF PHYSICIAN OR SUPPLIER INCLUDING DEGREES OR CREDENTIALS (I certify that the statements on the reverse apply to this bill and are made a part thereof.)

SIGNED _____ DATE _____

32. NAME AND ADDRESS OF FACILITY WHERE SERVICES WERE RENDERED (If other than home or office)

33. PHYSICIAN'S, SUPPLIER'S BILLING NAME, ADDRESS, ZIP CODE & PHONE #

PIN#   GRP#

(APPROVED BY AMA COUNCIL ON MEDICAL SERVICE 8/88)   **PLEASE PRINT OR TYPE**   APPROVED OMB-0938-0008 FORM CMS-1500 (12-90), FORM RRB-1500, APPROVED OMB-1215-0055 FORM OWCP-1500, APPROVED OMB-0720-0001 (CHAMPUS)

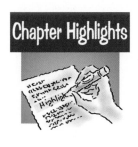

Chapter Highlights

- Most patients in a physician's office have some type of health plan.
- Payments from health plans provide the majority of most offices' income.
- Types of health plans include group, individual, and government-sponsored plans.
- Many physicians have contracts with managed care plans such as HMOs and PPOs.
- Each plan and type of plan has certain requirements about eligibility for payment of services.
- Your primary duty in filing claims is to do so in a timely and correct manner that will ensure maximum reimbursement for the office.

GLOSSARY

abandonment   when a physician withdraws from a contractual relationship with a patient without proper notification while the patient still needs treatment [Chapter 2]

accounting   the system and practice of setting up, maintaining, and monitoring an organization's financial records and activities, in order to keep track of its financial status and provide information for making business decisions; contrast with *bookkeeping* [Chapter 6]

accounts payable   the amount of money a business owes for goods and services it has received; the record of all debts a business has not yet paid; contrast with *accounts receivable* [Chapter 6]

accounts receivable   the total amount of money due to a business for goods or services it has provided; a record of all monies a business is owed; contrast with *accounts payable* [Chapter 6]

acute   coming on suddenly or quickly worsening; severe but lasting only a short time; contrast with *chronic* [Chapter 4]

adjustments   additions to or subtractions from an account (such as a patient's account) that do not result from charges incurred or payments received; for example, a subtraction due to a discount on the physician's fee or an addition due to the bank's return of a patient's check because there was not enough money in the patient's checking account to pay it [Chapter 6]

advance directive   a patient's statement of his wishes regarding future treatment in the event the patient is not able to communicate those wishes at the time [Chapter 2]

aging schedule   a record of accounts and balances in accounts receivable that have not been paid and how long each is past due [Chapter 6]

application   a software program that enables a computer to perform a specific function or task [Chapter 3]

assault   an attempt or threaten to touch a person without her consent [Chapter 2]

balance billing   billing the patient for the difference between the physician's charge and the charge allowed by the patient's health plan; this practice is prohibited by many managed care contracts. [Chapter 8]

battery the deliberate touching of a person, either directly or with an object, without his consent [Chapter 2]

bias an opinion that favors one thing, often unfairly or without a basis in fact or reason; prejudice [Chapter 1]

bioethics moral issues and concerns arising from advances in biology, medicine, and medical technology that affect people's lives [Chapter 2]

birthday rule a method for determining which health plan is first to pay when a patient is covered by two plans (for example, a child who is covered by the health plan of each parent); the plan of the policyholder whose birth month and day come first on the calendar is the primary plan and it is billed first. [Chapter 8]

bookkeeping the work of keeping a systematic record of an organization's day-to-day financial transactions; contrast with *accounting* [Chapter 6]

bookmark a saved link to a place on the Internet that allows a computer to access the place without the user having to enter its Internet address [Chapter 3]

capitation a method of paying for health care in which a managed care plan (usually an HMO) pays the physician a fixed fee for each member's care over a set period of time, no matter how much care the physician provides the member during that time [Chapter 8]

certification a voluntary process, usually involving testing, establishing that a person meets a certain standard of competency in a particular area [Chapter 2]

chronic lasting a long time or happening again often; contrast with *acute* [Chapter 4]

chronological order arranged in the order of time; in patients' charts, the oldest document is usually on the bottom and the most recent document at the top of the order. [Chapter 5]

civil law the branch of law that focuses on disputes between persons [Chapter 2]

clarification explanation; removal of confusion or uncertainty [Chapter 1]

clustering an appointment-scheduling system in which patients with similar problems, needs, or conditions are grouped in the same block of time [Chapter 4]

coinsurance the amount a health plan requires the policyholder to pay as her share of the cost of care, usually expressed as a percentage (for example, in an 80/20 plan, the insurance company pays 80 percent of the bill and the insured pays 20 percent as *coinsurance*); not to be confused with *co-payment* or *deductible* [Chapter 8]

communicable disease   a disease that can be passed from one person to another, either directly or indirectly [Chapter 2]

consent   agreement between a patient and a health care provider to perform a specific medical procedure [Chapter 2]

constellation of symptoms   a group or combination of clinical signs that indicate a specific disease process [Chapter 4]

consultation   the process by which a patient's physician obtains the opinion and advice of another health care provider regarding the patient's diagnosis, condition, or treatment [Chapter 4]

contract   an understanding between two or more parties in which each party agrees to do something [Chapter 2]

conventions   rules, practices, and methods that are generally accepted; in medical coding, the general notes, symbols, typeface, format, and punctuation that guide the coder to the most complete and accurate ICD-9 code [Chapter 7]

coordination of benefits   the process of determining the order in which health plans pay a patient's bill when the patient is covered by more than one plan, so that duplicate payment and overpayment will not occur [Chapter 8]

co-payment   a small sum of money that many health plans require a patient to pay at the time a medical service is provided; not to be confused with *coinsurance* or *deductible* [Chapter 6]

credit   a payment or other bookkeeping entry that reduces the balance due on an account; also, permission to pay later for goods or services [Chapter 6]

credit balance   any funds remaining in an account after the entire balance due has been paid; most credit balances result from overpayment and are especially possible when more than one payer (such as a patient and the patient's health plan) has been billed. [Chapter 6]

crossover claim   a billing that automatically passes from one health care plan to another for payment [Chapter 8]

cross-reference   a notation referring the user from one part of a list or other document to another place, in order to obtain more information [Chapter 5]

cursor   the movable position indicator on a computer screen that allows the operator to insert text in a document, open items on the screen, or drag items to a new location; cursor movement is controlled with the computer's mouse. [Chapter 3]

day sheet   a daily record of charges for patient services and payments received [Chapter 6]

deductible   a set amount of medical expenses that must be paid by the patient or policyholder before his health plan will begin paying; not to be confused with *co-payment* or *coinsurance* [Chapter 8]

defamation of character   making false or malicious statements about another person that damage the person's reputation [Chapter 2]

defendant   the accused party in a legal action; contrast with *plaintiff* [Chapter 2]

dependent   a spouse, child, or other person designated by an insured to be covered under her health benefits plan [Chapter 8]

discrimination   treating a person or a group differently from others [Chapter 1]

double booking   the practice of scheduling two patients for the same appointment period with the same physician [Chapter 4]

durable power of attorney for health care   a legal document that gives a person the authority to make medical decisions for a patient if the patient is not in a condition to make those decisions himself [Chapter 2]

electronic medical records (EMR)   information about patients that is recorded and stored on computer [Chapter 5]

encounter form   a preprinted form that lists ICD codes for diagnoses and CPT codes for basic services the office provides and has places to record charges for the services performed during an office visit, any payments received, and the balance remaining due [Chapter 6]

established patient   a returning patient who has previously been seen by the physician [Chapter 1]

ethics   guidelines for moral behavior that are set by religious beliefs, professions and other groups in society, and by individuals themselves [Chapter 2]

etiology   the causes of a specific disease [Chapter 7]

explanation of benefits (EOB)   the statement that is included with a payment from a health plan, indicating which dates of service and services the payment is for [Chapter 8]

expressed contract   a formal agreement, stated orally or in writing, between two or more parties; contrast with *implied contract* [Chapter 2]

fee schedule   a list of fees for specific services and procedures, either set by a health care provider or by a patient's health care plan [Chapter 6]

fee splitting the sharing of fees between physicians for patient referrals; generally considered to be an unethical practice [Chapter 2]

feedback in communication, the response to input from another person [Chapter 1]

flow sheet a form that allows information to be recorded in a graphic or tabular manner for easy retrieval [Chapter 5]

gatekeeper the name sometimes given a patient's primary care physician in some managed care plans, who must approve and make all referrals to other providers (The plan generally must approve these referrals too.) [Chapter 8]

grief deep or intense sadness or sorrow, usually resulting from a death or other personal loss [Chapter 1]

group the people who are covered under a master health plan sponsored by their employer or by some other organization to which they belong [Chapter 8]

hard copy a printed, paper copy of information from a computer; also called a printout [Chapter 3]

hard drive the device inside a computer that stores its programs and data files [Chapter 3]

hardware the physical equipment of a computer system, such as its monitor, central processing unit, keyboard, mouse, printer, and scanner [Chapter 3]

health care surrogate a patient's representative who makes health care decisions for the patient if the patient is unable to make them [Chapter 2]

Health Insurance Portability and Accountability Act of 1996 (HIPAA) federal law that set standards for the protection of patient information and for submitting claims to health insurance plans, and made other major health care reforms [Chapter 1]

implied consent informal approval from the patient to perform a particular task that is assumed from the patient's cooperation and attitude; contrast with *informed consent* [Chapter 2]

implied contract an agreement between parties, such as a patient and a physician, that is not stated but is assumed from the actions of the parties; contrast with *expressed contract* [Chapter 2]

incident report a form used by a health care organization to document an unusual occurrence to a patient, employee, or visitor [Chapter 3]

infectious disease a disease cause by the invasion of the body by microorganisms that multiply and damage body tissues or systems; some infectious diseases are also *communicable diseases* [Chapter 2]

informed consent a statement of approval from a patient, often given in writing, to perform a given procedure after the patient has been educated about its benefits and risks; also called *expressed consent;* contrast with *implied consent* [Chapter 2]

intranet a private internet that usually belongs to an organization, allows only its members access to its pages, and blocks other computer users who are not part of it [Chapter 3]

inventory a detailed list of the supplies, equipment, or other property that an organization has on hand; to make such a list [Chapter 3]

invoice a list of goods or services that have been provided, along with the prices or fees charged; a bill [Chapter 6]

itinerary a detailed outline for an upcoming trip or journey [Chapter 4]

key component a major factor on which the selection of a CPT-4 Evaluation and Management code is based [Chapter 7]

kinesics the study of body movements and facial expressions as a form of nonverbal communication [Chapter 1]

late effect a condition that results from another condition; for example, left-sided paralysis is often a *late effect* of a stroke. [Chapter 7]

legal guardian a person placed in charge of the affairs of a minor or an adult who is not mentally competent [Chapter 2]

legally required disclosures vents or conditions that health care providers must report to government authorities, despite the confidentiality of medical records and even without a patient's consent; examples include births, deaths, certain infectious or communicable diseases (such as sexually trans-mitted diseases), conditions that lead to suspicions of child abuse, and injuries that may have resulted from violent criminal acts [Chapter 2]

libel false and malicious written statements that damage a person's reputation or character; contrast with *slander* [Chapter 2]

malignant cancerous [Chapter 7]

malpractice injurious actions, improper actions, or neglect of a patient by a physician or other health care professional [Chapter 2]

medical ethics the values and guidelines that should govern decision making and behaviors in the delivery of health care [Chapter 2]

medical necessity a judgment that a certain service or proce-dure is appropriate based on the patient's diagnosis, symptoms, and sound medical practice; this decision is generally made by a third-party payer and is often required before it will pay for the service or procedure in question. [Chapter 7]

microprocessor   the chip or circuit inside a computer that enables the computer to interpret and carry out instructions from the programs running on it; the "brain" of the computer [Chapter 3]

minor   a person under the age of full legal responsibility, usually age 18 [Chapter 2]

modem   a device that allows a computer to send and receive data over a communications line such as a telephone line or cable television line [Chapter 3]

modifiers   letters and/or numbers that are sometimes added to a CPT code to give more information about the service that was provided or the procedure that was performed [Chapter 7]

morphology   the form and structure of an organism or of one of its parts [Chapter 7]

narrative   an account of events written in paragraph form [Chapter 5]

negligence   taking an action that a reasonable health care professional would not have, or not taking an action that a reasonable health care professional would have taken; in general, the failure to provide a proper standard of care [Chapter 2]

neoplasm   an abnormal growth of tissue, such as a tumor [Chapter 7]

outcome   the final result of the care and treatment a patient receives [Chapter 3]

packing slip   a form accompanying a shipment or delivery that lists the items enclosed [Chapter 6]

participating provider   a health care provider that has contracted with a managed care health plan to provide certain services to its members and in exchange for payment according to a preset schedule of fees; also see *preferred provider* [Chapter 6]

pathogen   a disease-causing microorganism [Chapter 2]

patient confidentiality   the protection of all information and data about a patient from those not authorized to have it [Chapter 2]

pediatrician   a physician who specializes in the care of infants, children, and adolescents [Chapter 1]

peer review   a process in which a health care professional's actions in a disputed case are reviewed and evaluated by a group of other health care professionals [Chapter 2]

petty cash a small cash fund kept on hand in an office to pay unexpected minor expenses [Chapter 6]

plaintiff the accuser in a legal action; contrast with *defendant* [Chapter 2]

posting recording individual financial transactions on a paper ledger or in a computerized bookkeeping or accounting system [Chapter 6]

precertification approval by a health insurance plan for a proposed treatment, consultation, or referral; many managed care plans require precertification and payment may be denied if it is not obtained. [Chapter 4]

preexisting condition a medical problem that existed before a health plan's coverage began; a health plan may limit coverage for problems the patient had before the plan's effective date. [Chapter 8]

preferred provider a physician or other health care provider who has agreed to provide services to an insurance plan's insureds for reduced fees; the plan usually offers financial incentives to its insureds to get their health care through its network of preferred providers; also see *participating provider* [Chapter 4]

prejudice an opinion or judgment about a person, group, or thing that is based on false information or ideas rather than on facts and reason [Chapter 1]

primary diagnosis the chief complaint or condition for which a patient is treated on a specific day or office visit [Chapter 7]

private pay the term used to describe someone who is paying a medical bill without the help of insurance or other third party payers [Chapter 6]

professional courtesy a discount on charges or fees that health care providers may sometimes give when treating health care professionals [Chapter 6]

program a set of coded electronic instructions that enables a computer and its user to perform a specific task, such as scheduling appointments or creating letters and other documents; also called an *application* [Chapter 3]

proxemics the study of how people use space in their interactions with others [Chapter 1]

referral the sending of a patient to another health care facility or physician, usually for special testing, treatment, or services [Chapter 1]

res ipsa loquitur a legal doctrine stating that things do not have to be explained beyond the obvious facts and that a person is presumed to be negligent if she had control of what caused an injury, even if there is no specific evidence of an act of negligence; Latin for "the thing speaks for itself" [Chapter 2]

res judicata   a legal doctrine stating that a matter settled in court cannot be raised again; it exists to protect parties in a case that has already been decided; Latin for "a thing decided" [Chapter 2]

respondeat superior   a legal doctrine stating that an employer is responsible for employees' actions performed within the course of their employment; Latin for "let the master answer" [Chapter 2]

scope of practice   the range of functions a health care provider is trained to perform; for a licensed professional, such as a physician or nurse, it is often set by law. [Chapter 2]

search engine   an Internet program that computer operators can use to do keyword searches for specific information on the Internet [Chapter 3]

slander   false oral statements that damage a person's reputation or character; contrast with *libel* [Chapter 2]

software   electronic instructions that allow users to interact with a computer or have it perform tasks for them; system software runs the computer itself, while application (program) software enables it to perform specific tasks [Chapter 3]

standard of care   how most other health care providers with similar training would have handled a patient's care under similar circumstances; the diagnosis and treatment process a health care professional should follow for a certain type of patient, illness, or clinical condition [Chapter 2]

stat   immediately or at once; an abbreviation of the Latin word *statim* [Chapter 1]

statute of limitations   a time limit for a certain legal action to be taken; for example, the maximum length of time in which a patient may file a lawsuit [Chapter 2]

stereotyping   holding beliefs about something that are based on beliefs about the group to which it belongs, without consideration that differences may exist among group members [Chapter 1]

straight digit filing   a chart-filing system in which patients' records are arranged in the numerical order of the patient numbers; contrast with *terminal digit filing* [Chapter 5]

streaming   a scheduling practice in which each patient is given one or more consecutive appointment slots, based on the time required by his or her needs [Chapter 4]

subject filing   arranging files by their title, grouping similar subjects together [Chapter 5]

surfing   the act of searching the Internet, especially by going from page to page by using electronic links (called *hyperlinks*) built into each page visited [Chapter 3]

terminal digit filing   a system for filing patients' charts in which records are filed according to the last two digits of the patients' numbers, then by the second-last set of two digits, and so on; contrast with *straight digit filing* [Chapter 5]

terminal disease   a disease that will cause the afflicted person to die and that is in its final stages [Chapter 1]

third-party administrator   a separate company or other organization that processes claims for a health plan [Chapter 8]

third-party payer   a health insurance plan or anyone other than the patient, the patient's spouse, or the patient's parent, who is responsible for paying all or part of the patient's bill [Chapter 4]

third-party payment   payment that comes from somewhere other than the patient or the patient's spouse or parent; most third-party payment comes from health plans. [Chapter 8]

tort   a wrongdoing that causes someone to suffer some type of injury or loss [Chapter 2]

triage   the sorting of patients into categories based on their level of sickness or injury, to ensure that those who most need attention are handled first [Chapter 1]

unbundling   the practice of submitting an insurance claim with several separate CPT procedure codes rather than a single code that covers all those services; sometimes done deliberately (and illegally) in order to obtain a larger payment [Chapter 7]

upcoding   billing more for a patient-care service than it is worth by selecting a CPT code that is higher on the coding scale than the service actually provided; this is an illegal practice. [Chapter 7]

wave scheduling   a flexible scheduling method in which patients are seen in the order they arrive, and which permits visit length to be adjusted for the patient's needs [Chapter 4]

workers' compensation   a health insurance program that pays for treating persons who suffer injuries or illnesses related to their jobs [Chapter 5]

FIGURE CREDITS

Illustrations in *Medical Assisting Made Incredibly Easy: Administrative Competencies* have been borrowed from the following sources:

Molle EA, Kronenberger J, Durham LS, West-Stack C. Lippincott Williams & Wilkins' Comprehensive Medical Assisting. 2nd ed. Baltimore: Lippincott Williams & Wilkins, 2005 (chapter 1, unnumbered figures 27 and 28; chapter 4, unnumbered figure 13; chapter 5, unnumbered figure 6; chapter 6, unnumbered figures 7 and 12; chapter 7, unnumbered figure 4; and chapter 8, unnumbered figures 7, 10, and 12).

INDEX

Page numbers in *italics* denote figures; those followed by a t denote tables.